Endometriosis - A Holistic Healing Guide

DISCLAIMER

This book is in no way offered as a cure for Endometriosis. It is here to offer guidance and advice on alternative therapies, tools and techniques that have helped the author. The therapies outlined in this book may assist you and are there to aid relaxation and stress symptoms. It is advised that you consult your GP should you wish to take up a therapy such as Yoga. Many alternative therapies do assist us and it is important that you remain in contact with your GP.

ISBN: 1-4196-0482-1

To order additional copies, please contact us.
BookSurge, LLC
www.booksurge.com
1-866-308-6235
orders@booksurge.com

TAMMY
LORRAINE MAJCHRZAK

ENDOMETRIOSIS —A HOLISTIC HEALING GUIDE

A HOLISTIC APPROACH FOR THOSE LIVING WITH ENDOMETRIOSIS, PMS AND ASSOCIATED SYMPTOMS

"A *book for every woman*"

2005

Endometriosis - A Holistic Healing Guide

CONTENTS

This Book Is Dedicated To Three Special People In My Life. Firstly, My Wonderful And Most Beloved Husband For Putting Up With My Search For Alternatives Over The Years And Giving Me The Confidence To Finally Publish This Book. Secondly, To My Father Who Has Sadly Passed Away But Who I Know Also Played A Big Part In Me Finally Publishing This Book. Last And Not Least To My Dear Mother Who Has Also Put Up With My Enthusiasm For Alternatives Over The Years! I Love You Very Much And Thank You For Supporting Me When At Times I Know I Have Been Very Difficult!

BRIEF INTRO

This book is about my personal experience of living with Endometriosis ("Endo") and how I have come to be pain free. I was not sure how this book would be received but I knew that the techniques I had used and are still using, benefited me greatly so I just had to put pen to paper. I was a little apprehensive initially about how I would put this book together, could I cram all the knowledge I had learned over the years into one simple book that would be easy to use, easy to follow and most important, would bring about positive changes.

This book is for all women across the world who may also suffer from Endometriosis, painful periods and discomfort at that time of the month that we are all familiar with. I hope that the pages to follow will benefit your life and health as they have mine. This book is a for those who feel frightened, out of control, worried, anxious, scared and my hope is that the techniques and advice in this book will go some way to offer you some support.

Endometriosis is now being more widely acknowledged as an illness and there are those who are in conflict whether it is an illness or a condition. Those who have this illness will know that their lives can be completely turned upside down on an emotional, physical and mental level.

As someone who is greatly interested in alternative therapies I have spent many years reading, trying & testing many products and techniques that bring harmony and balance to our mind, body and spirit. A great deal of what is written here comes from my own understanding of Endometriosis. Why I believe I have experienced the illness, my thoughts, feelings, literally 'my own experience'.

Later in the book I will briefly cover some of what I feel are possible explanations of why Endo occurs but one important thing to remember is that you don't blame yourself for having Endo. This is a negative attitude and it will not help you. You have to learn to be positive. Learning how to remain calm and bring balance to your life will help. When we are in control we are focused, when we are focused we have mental clarity. When we lose control, we lose focus, we lose interest, and we become ungrounded. We therefore need to take the journey to the inner self to find balance and focus and inner calm. It is hoped that this book will help you bring serenity and peace into your life on some level.

You might be thinking, "Well it's easy for her to say that, she hasn't got the same symptoms as me". Believe me I have suffered, I have been there, frightened and rolling about in agony not knowing what is going on inside of me and not understanding; which is equally as frightening as the pain itself. I have heard many stories, some quite horrific, from ladies who have got Endo. I have found that the greatest help has been to educate yourself and talk to others, share your experiences, learn from others, then we can perhaps begin to understand this illness.

I mentioned earlier getting in touch with the inner side of us. Many of us have lost touch with ourselves through no fault of our own. Getting in touch with our inner emotions and feelings really does help. The stepping-stones for this journey to the self are very small, but are very important. How can you begin to heal or deal with an issue, illness or problem if you don't know you! It is all so easy to reach out for painkillers and medication when what we should try to do is to find the root cause as to why our body is in pain. I am not saying here that we stop taking medication immediately that would not be a good thing but maybe looking at this illness in another light and trying to understand what is causing it.

Therapies and techniques such as grounding work, meditation and relaxation allow our body the time to rest and gives us a break from day-to-day activity. Meditation is a wonderful tool as it switches off the endless chitchat and chaos that goes on. We take a brief break from life as we allow our body and mind to relax and unwind.

My understanding as to why Endo might possibly occur

I wanted to highlight how important it is that we begin to look at this illness differently. It was through inner healing work and getting to know myself and listening to my body that I began to understand this illness a little better. I have listed below some ideas that have been put to me as to how Endo may possibly occur:-

- Genetics—our actual physical building blocks, tissues, muscle, bone marrow—basically the way we are made up

- Emotional issues

- Past trauma

- Outside pollutions/toxins in food etc (these may not be the main cause but will certainly add to symptoms)

- Abusing the body through poor diet

Conventional v Alternatives

Some will say that Endometriosis is not an illness that can be fully managed using alternative products and methods. Depending on your degree of pain, you will need to be seen by either your General Practitioner, Doctor or a Specialist Consultant. This I agree with to an extent as I have tried the conventional approach and have scars to show for this. I have to say that the alternative methods I have used have significantly reduced the pain and discomfort I was experiencing and I didn't get the same results from using any conventional medication.

At this point I feel it necessary to mention that I am not in support of only using conventional medication to assist Endometriosis. I have used contraceptives and for someone who is very in tune with her body I began to notice how some symptoms would begin to develop from using these medications so I decided to look at a more alternative approach. Many of the conventional medications offered to us dry up our body and interfere with the natural cycle. But for some of us conventional medication is the only way we know to deal with this illness so we need to approach this carefully. Not everyone is suited to alternative therapies. Not everyone believes these therapies can help them. But with a gentle approach and a little guidance we can learn from others.

Many people are not interested in alternatives. We have all had our fair share of bad experiences but there are many people, myself included who have found great relief and support from using alternatives. This is why I felt this book necessary to write. A favourite saying of mine on a light-hearted note is "the proof of the pudding is in the eating" and that is very true. What works for one person may not work for another but it is through personal experience and feeling that we know something is working well for us.

Yoga, for instance, as an alternative really can help as it works wonders with the human body. You will find therapies that don't agree with you but the therapies I use namely Yoga, meditation and healing techniques have helped to balance and calm me which is why I felt it necessary to want to share them with other fellow sufferers. The alternative methods detailed in this book show how we can use natural methods alongside conventional medication. You will realise that with regular practice with Yoga for instance, your symptoms may not be so severe and you may become less dependent on the conventional medications you may be currently taking. (*Please note this book is in no way offered as a sole alternative to conventional medication. I am simply showing you an alternative approach*).

So many individuals depend on the conventional medications that actually can be quite toxic to our system and bring many other symptoms on top of what you will already have! It is through my own experience that I have decided not to rely solely on conventional medication.

I have personally found that allowing my system to be free from toxins, including the conventional medications, drugs, etc has helped me to bring about a balance where my body can begin to heal naturally. You must remain in contact with your GP at all times as his/her opinion and guidance when suffering from Endometriosis is of vital importance. Through using alternative methods I have used qualified Alternative Practitioners and I would advise you to do the same. It may be wise to consult your GP if you wish to take up Yoga for example and ask if it is safe to do so. Yoga is very natural, but it is always best to check with your GP first.

What Therapies?

I have not included all Alternative Therapies. There are many that I have not tried which I am sure will be equally as beneficial. What I have included are those that I have personally used and that have given me the greatest benefits. The therapies mentioned are mainly those associated with Yoga such as breathing techniques, relaxation and de-stressing methods. As a qualified Yoga Practitioner I have kept to this therapy as it gave me positive results. One important factor is many of us don't spend time with ourselves. We rush about, doing this and that often for other people that we end up exhausted. Endo greatly affects energy levels so it is important to take time to relax and recharge our batteries. Learning to recognise when you are tired and need a rest is important otherwise we end up being short and irritable with others, and especially ourselves!

During relaxation and meditation our mind is switched off and it is in this kind of 'suspended animation', this quiet stillness of the mind that the body gets a break and is rested and rejuvenated. For Endo sufferers this quiet time is vital for healing. Alternative Therapies can assist us and bring benefits to health in many different ways. Over the years I have tried and tested hundreds of different therapies often to the dissatisfaction of my beloved Husband! Spending a great deal of money, time and effort. Some of the efforts fruitless, but as mentioned early, some have brought me much benefit.

I didn't want this book to be full of complicated names for postures so again I have simplified this for your ease of reference. Of course if you want to explore Yoga in more detail there are many excellent practitioners and products on the market that you can read about, watch on Video or DVD and learn from. It is often frustrating in this day and age to find the right thing that works. There is so much out there for us to learn, so much to try that I wanted to be able to put this into a book so that you didn't have to do the legwork! I have had the many trips to the Doctors, the tablets, injections and operations and although some of them helped I still felt out of control, frightened and did not know what was going to happen to me. I wanted to take back my life and be in control again as Endo can take hold of us and make us feel completely off balance. Often with Endo we feel as if our lives are not our own anymore. Many of us don't feel like the same woman and feel quite powerless. Wanting to just feel healthy and have our body working normal again.

Throughout my journey with Endo I remain in constant contact with my GP and my Consultant and at any time that I feel it necessary to visit them I do so. So I mention again that it is important that you remain in contact with your GP.

"You don't have Endo that bad so it's easy for you to say that these therapies work?"

Well I do have Endo! I did suffer and it was extremely painful and I suffered for many years. I managed to relieve myself from the many symptoms of this illness by learning about how the body works, what role toxins play in this illness and how we can heal using natural products.

A little exercise—Try this for starters!

This will only take a few minutes:

Sit somewhere where you are not going to be disturbed, turn the lights down and lie down if you wish, get comfortable. Now take your awareness inside of yourself. You can close your eyes if you wish. Now just begin to focus on how you feel right now with this illness. Is it controlling your life? Does it dominate everything you do, think, feel, say etc? If it does then you need to look at changing this and you can do this with some of the tools I have outlined in this book such as meditation, connecting with your inner self/inner healing and having a more positive approach instead of letting Endo take over you. Is this possible? You might ask - of course it is but it is up to you to make positive changes and you can do it. I did and it does involve a lot of changes in your life from looking at what you eat, your attitude to life, the people around you, at work, etc. Do you want this Illness to take over your life - a direct answer is probably 'Hell no'!

So what about Yoga and Endo?

Yoga balances our whole system working from the inside out. It brings clarity and stillness of mind. It rejuvenates and revitalises us. The benefits are just too numerous to mention. Yoga brings stability in many areas of life. When we find this stability we learn to cope better with whatever life throws our way. We slow down, we begin to listen to our bodies and notice perhaps for the first time, what is going on inside. Yoga specifically works and targets the Endocrine system. The Endocrine system plays a very important role in our body. It's message-sending hormones influence the operations of all of the body's tissues and organ systems.

This centralized role in controlling body functions is sometimes compared to that of the nervous system. But in general, the Endocrine System operates in a less rapid but longer-lasting manner than the nervous system, regulating slower processes, such as metabolism and cell growth. The nervous system's functions, on the other hand, are more immediate, such as the control of breathing and body movement. So you can see from this brief overview how important the Endocrine system is. Meditation is also important as in the quiet time of meditation and resting in postures we begin to switch off the monkey brain, the endless chit chat and begin to be at one with ourselves.

I have not outlined all Yoga postures, that would take a long time, as there are so many. I have concentrated mainly on those that work with specific "Endo hot spots" such as the hips, waist, and lower back, and postures that work to help bring that all important balance and alignment to body, mind and spirit. I have highlighted with the postures how they will benefit you and how they can assist you.

Take your time working with the postures. Become familiar with them and with time it will become second nature to practice. Do a little each day until you build up your confidence with the postures. With the Sun Salutation routine break the postures down one by one until you become familiar with them. The pictures will help.

If you are new to Yoga it is important that you don't over stretch and hurt yourself. There may be days when you don't feel like doing it; these are often the best days to practice! Be kind to yourself above everything else, and, if you have really off days then rest, it's as simple as that. Learn to listen to your body and know your limitations at this time. Work slowly and feel how your body feels after practice. Make it fun to do, make it your special time, time for YOU!

Some Initial Discomfort

When you first start practicing you may have some initial discomfort. This is only naturally as you may not have exercised for a while. Although Yoga is very natural if you are concerned about practising it is best to speak with your GP. Obviously you wouldn't practice just after an operation. But Yoga will help you to open up the body, and this should be a slow and gentle process initially until your body is used to the postures and you become more flexible.

I did experience a little discomfort when I started to practice. I didn't realise that the pulling pain and dull aches in my lower back were due to lots of adhesions that had formed because of Endo, all located in the pelvic area and lower back. It was only after having a Laparoscopy that I discovered what was causing this pain.

What is a Laparoscopy?

A Laparoscopy is usually performed as a minor operation during day surgery and is performed by a specialist consultant. The Laparoscopy gives the Consultant a direct internal view of the Peritoneal Cavity, Ovaries, outside of the tubes and the Uterus. The Laparoscopy itself is an instrument that resembles a very small telescope with a fibre optic system, which brings light into the abdomen. It is about the same size as a fountain pen and twice as long. An instrument to move the uterus gently out of the way during surgery will be placed in the vagina. Carbon dioxide (CO2) is put into the abdomen through a special needle that is inserted just below the navel. This gas helps to separate the organs inside the abdominal cavity, making it easier for the physician to see the reproductive organs during a Laparoscopy. The gas is removed at the end of the procedure. There can sometimes be discomfort after the minor surgery due to the CO2 gas. This does wear off after a few hours. It does feel a little like bad indigestion and is nothing at all to worry about!

Now where was I, (I seem to have got slightly sided tracked but I thought it best to briefly outline what a Laparoscopy was for those of you who perhaps don't know. Please remember I am not a GP so my knowledge may be somewhat limited). There are some very helpful websites that you can visit if you wish to learn more about Laparoscopy. I have just covered the basics for you.

Now back to Yoga.

I continued to practice Yoga and I must admit although a little discomfort was felt it did get easier as my body opened up and my hips released. It felt as if I was holding a great deal of stagnant energy in my pelvis.

If you have adhesions around the pelvic area, lower back and around the bladder, practice slowly. When you begin to exercise in these areas there is a little tenderness as the body begins to open up. In time you begin to free up these areas and your hips and groin will not feel so tense and stiff. Within a few weeks of practice you will notice a difference and your somewhat limited flexibility will improve day by day. Take your time and you will notice that your body will become more flexible and the energy will flow more freely throughout your being.

Illness often occurs when energy and toxins stagnate within our body. Yoga helps by working from the inside out, freeing up muscles, getting rid of tension and freeing the mind. When the body is tense so to the mind. I used to find it useful to have a hot shower or bath before practice to unwind and relax muscles. It helps your muscles to release a little. This isn't always necessary but to warm up before practice is important.

The importance of Water

The twisting, turning, stretching that Yoga brings all helps to eliminate toxins from our internal organs and muscles hence it is important to drink water to help flush the toxins out of your system. Many headaches and mood swings can be due to dehydration so make water your best friend. Opt for water instead of fizzy drinks. They will not ease dehydration. Water is the best option. It will also help your complexion and cellulite!

Not all the same

We are all different and each one of us will be at different levels of flexibility. Flexibility will come in time and with regular practice although this is not the key issue with Yoga. The body benefits from the relaxation alone, regardless of how far you can bend, stretch and twist. I am not saying the information in the following pages are going to heal you completely but what I will say is that they are tried and tested, simple practices that will aid you, but they have without doubt helped improve my life.

I believe that if we can truly express our experience from the heart, others can benefit. Some of you might be lucky enough to know how your Endo started but for the majority we don't know. We might not even know what is causing it and this in itself is very frustrating for us.

Our emotions and hormones are all affected by this illness. We often feel dirty inside, and so it is a natural response to feel moody, unloved, not being able to cope, feeling like you are losing your mind!

Looking Back

Thinking more on how my Endo possibly started one moment that seems pretty poignant was when I was about 21 sitting at home watching telly and suddenly having the most awful stabbing pain in the right lower side of my abdomen. Although the pain subsided after about an hour my Mother still insisted I call the Doctor to come check me out. The doctor could find no real cause for my pain and as the pain had almost disappeared there were no tablets prescribed and I was asked to rest. I had always had what I though were 'normal' periods, that is swollen belly, back pain and headaches, coupled with the insatiable hunger to eat anything and everything sweet!

As I got to say 24-25 they became a little heavier and a lot more painful but I just put this down to the fact that I was a woman and thanks to Eve we all had to endure this pain once a month! I had also started to become a little scatty in my brain and kept misplacing things and had terrible mood swings—the less said the better! I was completely out of balance! I knew that something was not right inside of me. It was almost as if I was completely off balance within my own skin and I thank my subconscious for helping me make the right decisions to get this checked out. My stomach always seemed bloated and sore, which I have since found out is nothing to do with Endo but intolerance to whole milk! I have been on skimmed milk now for 12 months and have a wonderful flat tummy and have lost 6lbs to boot! It's weird how something so simple as changing your diet can actually ease some of the symptoms that we blame Endo for!

Briefly –How I found out I had Endometriosis

So there I was on the bed having an internal when the GP hit a sore spot! He advised me there and then that I might possibly have Endometriosis. "Endo what"! I remember saying and was referred for a Laparoscopy to see what was going on. My appointment came for my operation. I went and had it done and remember feeling really oozy coming out of the anaesthetic. (If you have never had this done and are worried there is absolutely nothing to be worried about. It is a very common procedure). You have a needle placed in the vein in the top of your hand and you then feel a really funny sensation almost like someone put ice into your veins! It is not uncomfortable just such a strange feeling. In no time at all you are asleep.

I was really nervous about going under, as I did not understand where I would go if you know what I mean. Well I must say I woke up and felt like the world had been lifted from my shoulders. The 2—3 hours that I had been 'out of it' had given me such a peaceful rest! After the Laparoscopy the Consultant told me that I had quite a lot of adhesion sites and that this would account for my constant back pain and pulling sensations. I was advised to either go on some form of contraceptive to manage the pain and also to have some kind of surgery to remove the adhesions. It took me about 12 months to face up to the fact that I was going to have to take some form of medication to help me. I did not want to do this but as long as I was having my monthly cycle there was going to be pain, trauma and I just couldn't face it.

One evening after I had been doing one of my Yoga classes one of my students came up to me and we started talking and it came about that she had Endo. She mentioned to me that there was a new type of treatment that used an instrument called 'Helica'. I did not want the usual operation as I found that it was not for me and I had heard so many horror stories from women who had had operation after operation, bits removed (often when it was not necessary) and I just did not want to be in that position.

I went to see the consultant who carried out the Helica treatment, they used some kind of long-winded name for the type of surgery I was opting for but basically I was going to have the adhesions lasered off, rather than cut out (the Helica treatment is very gentle, non-evasive surgery and is gentle on the surrounding organs and tissues). I was advised to still go on some kind of contraceptive to help me to manage the monthly pains. I decided, against my better judgement! to go on Depo Provera. I only decided to take this because the Consultant had advised me that all the ladies he had treated for Endo who had been on Depo did not return for treatment and overall it became more manageable.

The reason for this as many of you will know is the Depo stops the monthly cycle and without this the Endo cannot grow/form and the adhesions die off—for some this is true, for others it doesn't help but I will continue - The Depo was great for pain management, no periods but the weight gain on Depo can turn people off it. I had to wait 8 to 10 months for my appointment so in the meantime I began the Depo Provera injections.

I was told that this did not always work for everyone and some individuals had experienced some quite bad side effects such as headaches, migraine, weight gain, mood swings etc whilst on the drug. After monitoring the pain using my pain management diary I could feel that my symptoms were getting better. The pulling pain had eased and life was a bit more bearable. The Depo Provera also stopped many of the symptoms associated with PMS such as headaches and nausea. Whilst on the Depo I found I was a little more tolerant with things, but became a little tearful 2—3 injections later.

The only problems I found on Depo is the weight gain, irritability and headaches eventually returned. I am usually about 56—58 kg (8 to 8 ½ stone) so my weight moving to nearly 9 ½ stone had an impact on me. Being relatively fit and lively, I felt each additional pound and I hated it. I had really noticeable Cellulite on my legs too, I had not had this before going on Depo. Seeing all these changes in my body made me want to change; I wanted to be normal again. The Cellulite was due to the toxins building up in my system, the foreign bodies that my body could not deal with). The decision—come off the Depo and see how I go. I felt clogged up and my head felt foggy as if I couldn't think straight. Then I realised that I was messing about with my natural internal body clock and this somehow didn't feel right and it certainly wasn't natural.

Needless to say I came off the Depo Provera and have promised myself never to taken anything like this again. Many women will swap and change contraceptive injections, pills etc over years and do not realise the damage they are doing to their own body. Read this book ***'Every Woman's Book' by Paavo Airola*** (ISBN0-932090-10-9) and you might be surprised to find what the contraceptives do to you. This is not to frighten you; on the contrary, it is to help you to look at your body from a more natural approach. Give the book a read, it's very eye-opening.

Most Doctors will advise us to take some kind of medication to help us to manage the symptoms better. I am in total agreement with this as long as we remain in control of what we are taking. If something does not agree with you then speak to your GP tell him/her your side effects, how you felt before, how you feel now and if you are not happy then try something else. I prefer to keep my system natural and it works for me and many other women.

I wish you well with your journey of discovery.

With love

Tammy Lorraine Majchrzak
AIYS (Dip. Yoga)

SECTION 1
WHAT IS ENDO—A BRIEF OVERVIEW

This is just a brief overview. There are many websites to visit, some of which are detailed at the end of this book, where you can find out more in-depth knowledge about this illness. (This is briefly what I have learned and just wanted to show an overview, keeping it short and simple.)

Many of us will have Endometriosis and won't even realise we have it. It is often referred to as the 'silent' illness that is we may have it but not necessarily know this as we all too often put the symptoms down to that time of the month and the usual PMS pains etc. Many of us find out we have Endometriosis purely by accident.

We may experience period pains that we cannot endure any longer, we may get headaches, outside of our natural cycle, unexplained bleeding, bloatedness, symptoms too much to bear. We take a trip to the GP and after a scan or internal examination are told we have Endo. I do believe there are a lot of women out there who suffer with Endo and still do not realise they have it. They will rely on pills from their GP to get them through each month. They won't look any further as they believe that it is just PMS! This is one of the danger zones with Endo. Many ladies that I have spoken to have had Endo and/or associated symptoms from being a teenager and as early as 11 or 12 years of age and only find out in their late 20s! The Endo has already done so much damage that they are often riddled with pain and symptoms that they cannot explain.

Endo brings many symptoms. I will list some common symptoms that many sufferers have experienced. I have gathered together some information kindly given to me by The Simply Holistic Society (SHE Trust). This is a brief overview of Endo and it's associated symptoms. Please note this list is not exhaustive, there are many other symptoms. I have highlighted the main ones to look out for if you suspect you might have Endo.

Endometriosis when broken down as follows, gives us the meaning of the Illness:

"End"—Greek word meaning ***inside***
"Metra"—Greek word meaning ***Uterus/womb***
"Osis"—Greek word meaning ***Illness, problem, something not right, abnormal happening.***

So we can see from the breakdown of the words what Endometriosis is about.

Endometrium is the tissue that lines the inside of the womb. It is believed that endometriosis occurs when cells from the Endometrium are found outside the womb, predominantly surviving near the uterus, bowel, bladder, ovary or fallopian tube. These cells then multiply, swell and break down, but they have no means of escape thus causing pain, inflammation, adhesions and cysts. Endometriosis scarring and adhesions/cysts can be found in many places—to name but a few:

Ovaries
Tubes
Outside Bowel
On ligaments supporting pelvis, hip etc
Inside Bowel
Pouch of Douglas (located at base of spine near the Perineum - between vagina and anal passage!)
Bladder
Uterus
Umbilicus
Vagina

Adhesions and cysts have also been found in the lungs and other parts of the body and it has also been know for male subjects to have had this Illness so it is not necessarily linked directly to females. These cases are rare but it just shows you how diverse this Illness is.

Some more symptoms/associations with Endo:

- Infertility: between 30 and 40% of women with endometriosis are infertile;
- Constant and extreme pain;
- Social isolation because it is too painful to move: sometimes simply getting out of bed is too hard, let alone leaving the home. Holding a conversation often uses 'too much energy' so the sufferer remains isolated, sometimes bedridden and *alone;*
- Depression: many feel loss of quality of life due to ongoing pain and discomfort;
- Breakdown of relationships due to the stress caused by the condition/partner not understanding;
- The inability to work and thus financial hardship. The National Endometriosis Society often do surveys and the last time they surveyed its members who had had time of work - the average number of days take off per year was 45 days a year.

I don't think anyone fully understands why this Illness occurs. We know that we have to change the way that it is dealt with to stop women undergoing unnecessary surgery, anguish and heartache.

As women this is unpleasant as it is but to have an illness that brings us so much pain and problems is unbearable at times. Our monthly cycle is a very natural occurrence. It is when our body flushes out toxins and prepares for bringing a child into this world. If we wish to that is. When this cycle is upset and painful it creates a great many emotional problems for us. Many Endo sufferers opt for stopping this natural cycle because they just cannot bear to live with the pain. Is this really the only option? For me this seems quite sad.

As a woman having a period is a natural process. So when we stop this process, and for some at a young age, seems very unfair and unnatural. This is where I believe more problems occur as we interfere with the body's natural cycle. The body has many natural rhythms and cycles and stopping or interfering with this brings many complications.

I feel that education is the key and I wanted to highlight some points to look out for. If you experience any of the following then you might want to look into this further with your Doctor. It is not to say you have Endo but it is better to discuss any concerns with your Doctor:

- ***If you suffer from pain during or after a period;***
- ***You rely heavily on medication to get you through your period;***
- ***You find intercourse painful and try and avoid it;***
- ***You have infertility problems;***
- ***You suffer from lower back pain or discomfort outside of your period;***
- ***Your abdomen is unusually bloated;***
- ***Stabbing pains, throbbing sensation and discomfort around the abdomen/ovaries;***
- ***Discomfort around the bladder and/or Uterus;***
- ***Pains and aching on urination;***
- ***Pain and discomfort when emptying the bowels! Hard stools, constipation (many Endo sufferers may also experience IBS and more often than not complications around the bowel area);***
- ***Blood and discharge outside of the period present in urine and faeces;***
- ***Nausea and sickness accompanied with headaches;***
- ***Listlessness, anxiety, depression;(this can be linked to normal PMS symptoms but severe cases are also associated with Endo);***
- ***Pain and discomfort that you cannot tolerate without taking medication;***
- ***Severe mood swings—often caused by PMS but severe cases can also be linked to Endo. It also denotes a hormonal and mineral imbalance in the body;***

You might have other pain and symptoms that I have not included above. If you feel that something is not right then please speak with your GP. It is better to be safe. If you have 2 or more of the above symptoms it is likely that you may have Endo. To rule this out and to be sure you should see your GP. Tell them you are concerned that you might have Endo. They will know how to check and advise you.

I had quite a few trips to the Doctor and with my symptoms and history of abdominal pain etc and they did deal with it very professionally. But I have to stress that *I was the one to initially take control of my situation, I went to the GP, I pushed for further investigations*, and this is an important point to remember. Be honest with your GP and tell them exactly how you feel, what your symptoms are etc, and go from there. If you do suspect you have Endo my advice is read up on it and educate yourself about it. At least then you can have a greater understanding instead of being in the dark. It only takes a quick visit to your GP to ask about this and get checked out. That is not to say everyone should go and get checked out but those who experience pain and discomfort that is often outside of their normal cycle and PMS. Your GP will not be able to diagnose there and then if you have Endo. He/she will probably put you forward for an internal examination.

A Laparoscopy usually follows an initial consultation & internal by your GP or chosen Consultant. There is nothing to worry about and the Laparoscopy will help to find out what is causing your pain. One of the main issues with Endo is that as women we want to be healthy and especially down below! We want to function normally without any problems. Endometriosis has a great impact on the way we think and feel about ourselves. Our emotions are greatly affected. We don't feel all woman and this is very painful both emotionally and physically. The greatest thing to share is the knowledge that something has worked or is working for us. To pass that on to others to help them. We are all unique individuals and we need to find that all important balance and we can with a little knowledge and a little help.

Some people describe Endometriosis as 'some slight discomfort and bleeding outside of the normal period'. Now as many of us know it is far more involved than this. Endo affects us emotionally, physically and mentally and for some spiritually as we ask 'what have I done to deserve this illness?' Do not blame yourself. This is not a good thing and brings more negativity into your life. Endometriosis is a very complex illness. Visit websites that have chat rooms and talks where you can see just how much pain many women all over the world are in. So to hear that it 'brings only slight discomfort' is greatly underestimating this illness. Many women are frightened. They don't know what is going to happen to them and they don't know where to turn. I ask that you take each day at a time and learn to keep a pain/symptoms diary when you start your new *regime* of fitness that may involve yoga, meditation, any therapies you choose. It is important to *pain manage* with the help of a diary so you can monitor how you are doing and if anything is changing for the better. There is a diary at the end of this book that you can utilise. They really do help. Especially if your bleeding cycle is all over the place and you want to monitor your cycle more closely.

SECTION 2
POSITIVE MENTAL ATTITUDE

I mentioned earlier that Endo often makes you feel out of control. Your hormones and emotions seem to be on an endless roller coaster ride. You might have good days but they are very few and far between. You can get on top of this and you can start to be more positive. It takes more energy to be negative so work that out for yourself! Positivity can be a powerful tool. If you constantly say negative things to yourself such as;

- I feel so depressed today;
- I need to shout and argue as I feel lousy;
- I feel fat, ugly;
- I can't cope with this Illness anymore it is really making me depressed;
- What's the point of it all;
- There is no one to talk to;
- You can't help me with your ideas, you don't have Endometriosis, and how can you possibly understand;
- I must have done something wrong to get this Endo it is so unfair;
- I am useless and I don't feel like a woman at all;
- It is ok for me to shout and be nasty to people, that is how I feel inside and they have to accept that;
- I feel dirty inside and that makes me feel dirty outside, I hate myself;
- It is better not to exercise as when I do it is painful;

All this negativity creates a dark cloud around you. This dark cloud will bring along dark negative energy and this is not good. I see many people, not only those who suffer with Endo but in today's society, walking around with chips on their shoulders and dark gloomy faces. They seem to have the world on their shoulders and life has been so hard for them. If they would only begin to be more positive. It is all about how we think and how we are, it's all about *turning it around—turning the negative into a POSITIVE.*

This is very important to remember. It may take us many years to ***become*** who we are today and it can be very easy to make little changes that can benefit us greatly. Positive thinking works—how do I know? Because I apply it to my life everyday. Of course I don't walk around like Mary Poppins full of happiness all the times, we are all human and are bound to have our off days. What I am talking about is the conscious awareness of how we think day in day out, and what effect it has on our body, mind and spirit.

What does help is changing your attitude to illness and try to find a way of feeling positive about your situation. Many of us are in a great deal of pain. How can thinking differently take the pain away?

Well why don't you give it a go and you may be pleasantly surprised by the outcome. Being kind to yourself is vital.

- I can deal with this, there are others who are worse off than I am;
- My pain is bad today but instead of sitting around I am going to take a walk and get some fresh air and feel alive;
- I have not got much energy today but I guess my body needs to rest;
- Maybe there is no miracle cure but I can do something about this illness and I can start now;
- I will open myself up to new ways and new ideas;
- I am going to leave the old me behind and start fresh, start to be positive;
- I know I have this illness but I can cope with it, it won't get the better of me;

You may be saying right now "yeah right, like that's going to work"; actually yes it does work if you learn how to apply this positivity, this turning around in your everyday life. One symptom I have found that is very common amongst us is ***depression***. We often feel very dark and gloomy and sometimes we just don't want to carry on. The only person who can really help us out of these dark times is our self.

We need to begin to be positive about this illness. I don't mean we accept it and just suffer, I mean that we start to become positive about how we can change our lives for the better and begin to make small subtle changes that can help us. I have searched high and low, and believe me I mean searched, for hints, tips, tools or just something that could help me to manage. I have also learned to turn my own life around focusing on the positives rather than the negatives and although not easy initially you can learn to manage your life better by removing the negatives.

Here's a little tip for an instant boost from Nature. It's wonderful and it's free! Stare at the sun between the hours of 8am in the morning up to 1pm in the afternoon with your eyes closed. Only for 5—10 minutes. The energy and light of the sun begins to work on the iris (eye) and this energy and warmth penetrates the nerves in the eye and this follows all the way throughout the body and has an affect on the Pineal Gland and Endocrine System. You may see a pink colour or vibrant colours as your eyes soak up this wonderful energy! It is important that you only do this between 8am and 1pm, as the sun's rays are not too hot at this time. It is also linked to the internal body clock so the timing is important. Try it, it's very invigorating.

You can also use visualisation techniques, which are outlined later on in this book. A good tip is to tell yourself that "*just because it is dark outside does not mean I have to be dark inside*"! There is often a simple explanation for the way we behave and there is always another way to 'be'. One important tip—if you have done something that you are not particularly proud of for instance you chastised the cat or pushed the dog or shouted at the boyfriend, hubby, child because you were in a bad mood—forgive yourself, say to yourself:

"I forgive myself for acting in this manner, at the time I wasn't feeling to good"

Forgiveness is also a very powerful tool so learn to use it and apply it to any situation you are experiencing or have experienced in the past, forgiving not only yourself but others. You might want to apologise to your loved ones for acting in this manner to! It all helps to keep peace and tranquillity in your environment and you may learn to like forgiveness and apply it more often to your life. Those who share our life don't have Endo; maybe you need to explain to them that sometimes you have off days.

They don't have to put up with moods, bad tempers, etc but if you were to explain properly they may be a little more understanding. I have found that the longer you focus on the illness the more control it actually has over you. "That's easy for you to say", umm no it's not actually but again I have learned these techniques and I feel better in myself if I don't dwell on the fact that *I have Endometriosis.* I don't allow it to be a prominent factor in my life and it certainly does not take up my every waking moment. Yes I have an illness, yes I am living with it, but no I won't allow it to dominate my life. People with very serious and life-threatening illness have found great benefits and a reduction in symptoms from being more positive.

SECTION 3
THREE KEY TOOLS

PRANAYAMA, MEDITATION & VISUALISATION (PMV)

Forget PMS and think PMV! I have found that Pranayama (breathing exercises), Meditation and Visualisation to be very valuable tools. They help us to relax and tune into our inner core.

How do these practices benefit me?

Endo makes us feel ungrounded at times. Trying to cope with the pain, headaches etc can leave us feeling very drained of energy. We get ourselves all stressed out, panicky, nervous, anxious, worried etc—this just adds to the already ungrounded feeling and can be frightening at times. We are human beings we need familiarity, we need routine, and most of all we need to be *grounded.* So we need to bring back focus, grounding and learn to centre ourselves. Relaxation and meditation work wonders—bringing us down, making us calm. The breath is the key to relaxation and whilst performing healing sessions I have noticed how a person begins to relax almost instantly whilst focusing on their breath and the pattern of breathing. These techniques don't cost you anything and you can do them in the comfort of your own home.

Many of us don't breathe properly; believe it or not it's a fact. We tend to breathe into the top of our chest and this in itself can create problems over a long period of time. Learn to breathe deep down to your stomach/abdomen. It should be a gentle natural process, not over emphasised and you should feel comfortable. Obviously we can't do this 24/7 but if we learn correct breathing techniques and can apply it each day whether it be our own 10 minute relaxation and meditation before bed or when we have some spare time, or whether we practice it sitting at our desk at work, sitting tall and breathing into the stomach. It is simple to apply and takes no time at all. Over the next few pages I will introduce you to some basic visualisations and some basic breathing techniques. Should you wish to work with this on a higher level then my advice would be to visit your local yoga teacher/meditation centre and ask them for further advice.

There are books, CDs, DVD and other materials that can help you. There are more complex breathing techniques and if you wanted to practice these it should best be done under supervision of a trained yoga practitioner until you become familiar with them. You will see that visualisation is a kind of meditation in itself and also uses breathing so these 3 vital tools are all utilised in the following practices. The importance of these three techniques cannot be over stated so please try and use them as often as you can.

Pranayama (Breathing Exercises)

I cannot stress the importance of this with aiding Endometriosis. Breathing practices not only calm us but they help our stress levels and calm the mind. It is through breathing that we can help our body to heal. I mentioned briefly earlier that many of us do not breathe properly. To learn how to breathe properly again is not difficult.

Have you ever watched a baby breathe? Well next time you get the chance spend a few minutes just watching how they breathe. Their abdomen is fully utilised as they breathe deep down to the stomach. Filling the lungs completely and it is a pure and natural process. Watch and learn and you can then begin to do this yourself.

Whilst teaching in classes I often found that many students could not believe how over the years they had really let their breathing go! By that they meant that they had not really taken any notice of how they were breathing and how this process really had an impact on health. In this book I am only covering basic breathing techniques. Introducing you to some gentle practices, which will reunite you and your breath. It's amazing how through only a little practice each week we can greatly improve our lung capacity and overall health. I will cover these practices a little later on.

Why Meditate?

When we meditate or use a visualisation exercise our breathing relaxes as our mind switches off from all the worries of the day and we begin to ***focus*** on the breath. Our breathing is natural and there is a release, almost like someone turned a screw in our head and let all the steam out. This switching off of our thought pattern through focussing on the breath stops the endless chitchat that often goes on in our heads and gives us a rest.

Many people don't understand that meditation can actually be very easy and the easiest method is to use your natural breathing pattern *(as outlined in breathing exercise 1).* This has a profound impact on the chemicals in the brain and again begins to relax the mind. I won't get too scientific here, as that would be totally out of character for me! I want to point out how meditation benefits the body in so many ways from slowing down the heart rate, relaxing the mind and bringing us a kind of balance and harmony from deep within. I mentioned earlier about that quiet time that our body needs.

It really is important to allow our body and mind to experience this quiet time. This is when we let go, are neither awake nor asleep but in a state of peaceful bliss, where are mind, body and spirit can unite, we rest and the body begins to heal (this peaceful bliss is called ***Yoga Nidra*** a kind of suspended animation! When you are neither awake nor asleep—suspended bliss! Many of us are not familiar with our breath. We just breathe and we don't really take any notice of it.

Isn't the human body a wonderful thing. It does all these things day in day out, year in year out and we are often not even aware of it! We live day in day out and don't really take any notice of it but it is a wonderful tool that we can use to help us. I will later introduce you to a basic breathing exercise to bring awareness to the natural process and helps us to begin the journey of ***tuning in*** and ***focusing*** on our body.

What is Visualisation?

When we begin visualisation practice we are taming the mind. We begin to see things with our mind's eye or third eye and this can help with psychic development. Many have benefited from visualisations involving surrounding yourself with peace and tranquillity, lotus blossoms, golden lights, music, birds, peace and harmony. Water visualisations are also very beneficial as they bring us tranquillity.

In the beginning you may find it difficult to stay with the visualisation. When you become familiar with the routine you can do it automatically, that is without the aid of tapes and words, instructions etc. You will become familiar with your inner temple, your inner peace and will be able to visit there whenever you wish.

The beauty with visualisation is when you become familiar with using it you can be anywhere in the world, be anyone you chose, do anything that pleases you and brings you peace. It's a great technique.

SECTION 4
SEATED POSITIONS FOR MEDITATION & RELAXATION

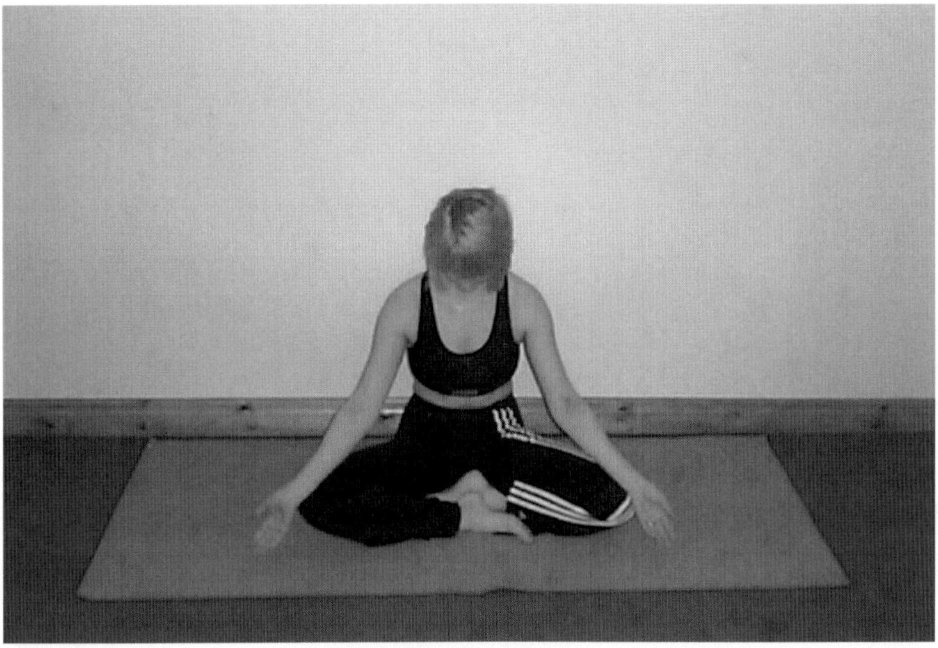

Seated Posture

There are many different seated postures you can use. The aim is to feel comfortable as you may be sitting from 5 to 20 minutes. The seated position shown above is one I use most frequently as it allows my back to be tall and my chest to open up allowing the air to flow through unrestricted. This is called *Virasana* in Yogic terminology but I don't want this book to be overcomplicated with long names for things you probably won't use! Find a seated position that you feel most comfortable in. Many choose the basic seated positions such as:

- Sitting crossed legged (basic position)
- Sitting on top of heels, knees bent, buttocks resting on heels. Spine tall.
- Half lotus—one leg crossed gently on top of the other.
- Full lotus—both legs crossed high at the groin so the legs are locked in a cross over position

If you cannot manage to sit on the floor you can use a cushion, or pillow. You can also use a chair to sit tall if you cannot manage the above-seated postures. It does not matter how you are sat, the emphasis must be on the back tall, shoulders lowered and rested, and chest open so the energy (breathe/prana/life force) can flow unrestricted. If you sit round shouldered, crouched over and body closed your breath will not flow freely. A good Yoga mat will help and they are not pricey. You can always use a warm cosy blanket to sit on. This will protect the knee area if sitting cross-legged.

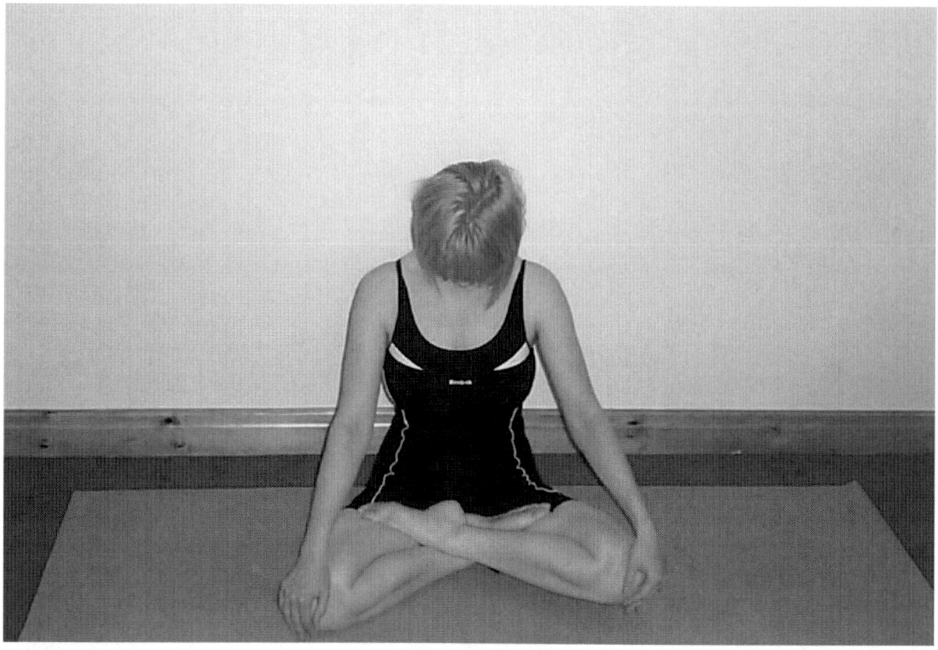

Full Lotus

The seated postures help to bring a fresh blood supply to the hip, groin, pelvis and reproductive organs. When you sit in these postures for a short while it can really benefit you. As the hips and groin relax, the lower back also relaxes, the hips open and relax. This can ease tension and relax muscles in the lower regions. To sit still with eyes closed for a short while can shut out the world for a brief moment. Try it, it really does help.

Don't rush to sit a certain way or sit in an uncomfortable manner. You will in time find a way to sit that suits you. You can just sit back on your heels if you cannot manage the above, or be seated on a chair if you cannot manage a seated posture. Be sure to sit up straight as this allows the energies to flow better through the entire body. If you crouch over you restrict air and energy flow (Prana). With regular practice you will find any initial discomfort will gradually ease.

SECTION 5
VISUALISATION EXERCISES

BRINGING IN THE SUN

We all need the sun, take flowers, trees and animals, they all need the sun and we do to. Think what a flower does if left in the dark, without water and sunlight it cannot survive. We are not so different. This visualisation is very simple. You can do this exercise either sitting down or lying down on the bed or floor whichever suits you. (*Words in italics—in case you might want to record on tape for later use).*

Always begin with the focus on the breath, entering the nostrils on the inhalation and leaving them on the exhalation.

Close your eyes, not tight, just so the eyelids are closed slightly and gently touching.

Now take your awareness to just outside the tip of the left nostril. Focus here as you begin to inhale though the nostrils.

Inhaling—the abdomen gently rises

Exhaling—the abdomen gently falls back naturally

Don't harness the breath, let it be natural, breathing in, the chest expands and following the breath deep down to the abdomen as it gently rises) holding the breath for a second or two

Then exhaling—watching the abdomen gently fall back to its natural position, exhaling all of the air out of the lungs, and begin exhaling, natural breathe...

Repeat this process for a few more breaths, become familiar with the rhythm of breathing and don't harness the breath, let it be natural, you are observing, watching the process, almost standing aside and watching how it happens naturally with no conscious effort.

(At any point or if you feel that your out of breathe, stop the practice and revert to normal breathing feel that your body wants to take in a really big breathe, let it happen, this just means that your body needs more energy that's all).

As you inhale imagine vibrant, fresh energy filling every part of you, every cell, every muscle, every part of you from the top of your head to the tips of your toes

Now bring your awareness to the top of your head and imagine the sun here, bright, energising sun at the crown of your head, it feels really warm and it is real bright energy.

On your next inhalation imagine the sun is right at the top of your head, shining down, bring the sun energy through the crown of your head and visualise it moving through your body filling you up with vibrant, fresh energy, that revitalises every cell in your body, it is a wonderful, piercing light that fills you with positive sun energy.

Still inhaling you bring this energy down to your stomach area and feel it lighting up with the sun's warmth.

As you exhale visualise all the negative stale energy in your stomach floating down past your legs and feet and disappearing into the ground.

Inhaling—bring the sun energy into the body, visualise the sun, inhaling (deepen the inhalation now, filling up your energy reservoir with positive light energy from the sun, notice now the lungs expanding with this energy and moving down to the stomach.

Exhaling the stale negative energy down away from your body.

Continue inhaling.........exhaling...inhaling...exhaling.

You can continue with this practice until you feel completely rejuvenated. You can work on deepening and lengthening the breath, but remember do it so it is comfortable. You should never hold onto the breath so that it is uncomfortable, it is always a natural process. If you want to lengthen the inhalation do so only as it is comfortable for you, you can use this technique:

In, 2, 3, 4, out 2, 3, 4, in 2, 3, 4 out 2, 3, 4

And work with lengthening as you become familiar and comfortable:

In, 2, 3, 4, 5, 6 out 2, 3, 4, 5, 6 etc.

The way we breathe has a great impact on the way we use our minds! It's true, if we are calm and relaxed and feel peaceful our breath is very quiet and it can feel like we are not breathing at all as the motion is so relaxed and natural. If we are angry or upset then our breathing is heavy, loud and out of its natural rhythm. If we are anxious and our head is whirling round because we are worried our breathing will reflect this and we have to take big breaths in case we hyperventilate. Get the picture? Next time you are fed up, worried, nervous, angry, upset etc tune into your breathing and see what is going on.

Breathing exercises can be done seated or lying down (corpse pose).

<u>If sitting:</u>

Cross-legged, Half Lotus, Full Lotus whichever is comfortable. Your back needs to be straight and see that you are not bent forward. This will be uncomfortable after only a few breaths. You must feel at ease, sitting tall and comfortable. Try and feel centred. This will help you relax whilst sitting and practising the exercise. Drop the shoulders and bring the chin gently into the notch in the chest, not all the way but just enough to feel the back of the neck lengthen, creating space.

IF YOU HAVE A BAD BACK AND ARE UNABLE TO SIT UNAIDED THEN USE A CHAIR AND MAKE SURE YOU SIT TALL WITH YOUR FEET TOUCHING THE FLOOR AND DROPPING THE SHOULDERS SO YOU DON'T HOLD TENSION THERE.

If lying down:

Find a quiet, comfortable place on a mat on the floor or even on the bed. Allow your feet to gently flop out to the sides, lift your head up gently and look towards your feet, you should feel centred, that is each side of the body feels balanced. If not then shuffle about until you feel balanced. Allow the arms to be about 2—3 inches from the sides of the body, palms facing towards the ceiling and begin to let yourself unwind.

SECTION 6
SIMPLE BREATHING TECHNIQUES

Exercise 1

Find your comfortable position before you start any meditation, visualisation or breathing. For this simple exercise we are sitting so find your comfortable seated position. Remember to sit tall, bringing the chin gently into the little notch in the chest, bring it towards not right on it! This just opens up the back of the neck. Shuffle about a bit to find comfort otherwise you will get lower back strain and feel uncomfortable. When you feel ready then you begin. When inhaling do so through the nostrils—if you have a cold then you can't obviously! So use the mouth but the best benefit is when using the nose to inhale) (you might want to tape the bits in italic!)

Now we begin the practice:

Finding your comfortable position, eyes gently closed, not tight, take your awareness to just outside the tip of the left nostril.

Take a deep INHALATION—deep down to abdomen—(notice as you inhale the abdomen gently rises)

Ready to exhale (notice as you exhale the abdomen falls back naturally)

As you exhale—imagine all the stagnant energy leaving the body, and the body itself relaxing with every exhalation, relaxing you deeper, further…

Inhaling deeply, through the nose, following the breath deep down to the abdomen, again it gently rises

When ready, begin Exhaling—all the stagnant energy leaving the body, as you fully empty the lungs…

Inhaling again, natural breathe, natural process, filling the body with energy, vibrant energy, you follow the breath on its journey deep down into the abdomen, again it gently rises…

Exhaling when you are ready, slowly, controlled not rushed,

One inhalation and one exhalation complete 1 cycle.

Do this for 10 cycles noticing with every exhalation how relaxed you feel. If you nod off, so be it!

Finish off with a deep breathe in, and exhale.

Breathing Exercise 2

ALTERNATIVE NOSTRIL BREATHING 1 & 2 - (with retention)

There are many different breathing practices in Yoga. Some of them are more complicated so we are going to keep it simple. As with all practices there needs to be some awareness made to contraindications. Some people because of their current health issues may not be able to perform some breathing techniques but overall with simple breathing practices such as these there is usually nothing to worry about.

Contra-indications:

Do not attempt to hold the breath if you suffer from any of the following:

- Heart problems, such as Angina, previous heart conditions etc
- Epilepsy
- High Blood pressure

With some conditions such as Diabetes and Low blood pressure, breathing practice does benefit immensely but again exercise caution. If at any time you feel uncomfortable then stop the practice. These are simple breathing techniques and have no risks to health.

Let's begin:

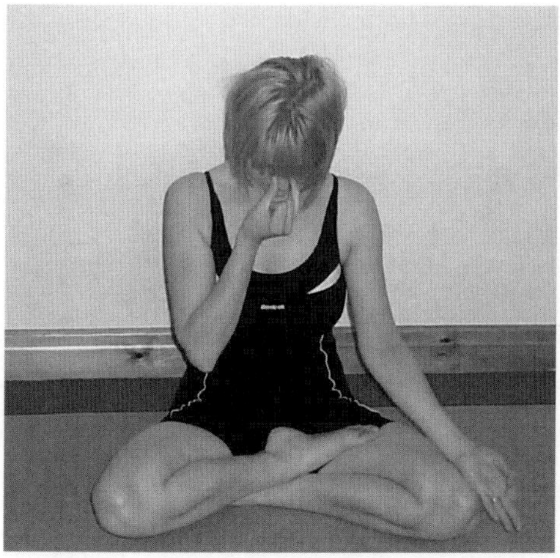

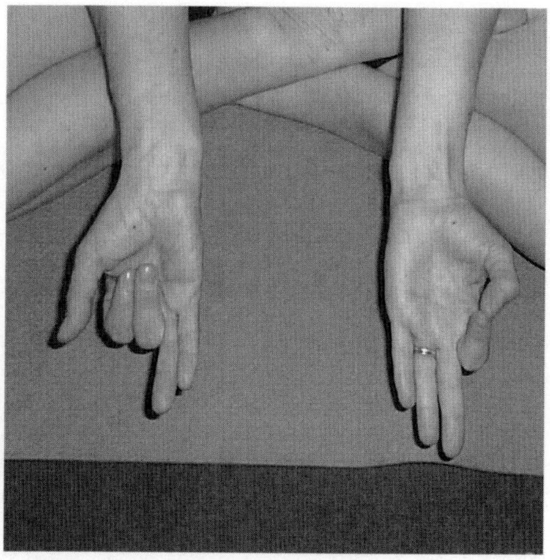

Alternate Nostril Breathing & Hand Mudra

- Find your comfortable seated position:
- Taking the left hand and placing it on top of the left knee, thumb and first fingertip touching making a circle shape (this is called a hand mudra and is said to symbolise the self-uniting with the

Universe—see images above). The knuckles of the left hand should rest on the knee, other fingers of left hand outstretched or passive whichever you feel most comfortable with.

- The right hand taking the first and second fingers either into the palm or resting above the nose, between the eyebrows (third eye point), the thumb rests against the outside of the right nostril, just passive, the 3rd and little finger resting outside the tip of the left nostril. Gently close your eyes. You don't have to but it is easier to focus internally and feel the exercise working from within. If your eyes are open you don't focus internally as much and the mind does tend to wonder. If we shut the outside world out simply by closing our eyes gently, we focus our awareness internally.

- Begin by gently pressuring the third and little finger to close off the left nostril.

- Inhale through the right nostril - at the end of the inhalation, block off the right nostril with the thumb so now both left and right nostrils are closed.

- Holding onto the breath for a second or two then release the left nostril only as you control the exhalation.

- At the end of the exhalation, inhale through the left nostril.

- At the end of the inhalation, block off the left nostril so now again both nostrils are closed, holding the breath again for a second or two, only as long as is comfortable, don't harness the breath.

- Then releasing the right nostril as you slowly (and controlled) exhale.

- Then releasing both nostrils as you inhale and exhale as normal, naturally.

This completes one round.

<u>Let's simplify:</u>

- Close off left nostril;

- Inhale through the right nostril;

- At the end of the inhalation, block off both nostrils (retain breathe in);

- Hold breath 1, 2 - release left nostril only - control the exhalation;

- At end of exhale, inhale through left nostril;

- At the end of inhale block off left nostril both nostrils blocked;

- Hold 1, 2 - release right nostril as you exhale;

- Release both nostrils as you return to normal breathing;

(If you have a cold or sinus problems you may find that your nostrils are blocked. If this is so do not practice. Wait until the nostrils become clear otherwise you will strain).

Benefits of this practice

- Calms the mind;
- Clears the head;
- Helps clear the sinuses;
- Helps Asthmatics as can help to regulate breathing;
- Regulates the breath/breathing process;
- Helps with panic attacks and anxiety;
- Reduces stress, as you focus internally;
- Can help you to think straight;
- Excellent for building up the lungs/capacity, cleansing and clearing cobwebs and stagnant energy.

You may experience a 'popping' sensation in the nose. This is freeing up energy, stagnant energy and clearing the airways. It is nothing to worry about. It is evidence that the energies are freeing up and working. It can be very releasing. With regular practice you will be able to do this as second nature without notes and with no conscious thought. Remember to take a few moments after practice to notice how you feel. Work slowly with the breathing practice. Over time and with familiarity you will be able to work on lengthening the holding of the breath. When practised correctly it should feel natural and rhythmic. You may experience a cooling sensation in the third eye area/behind the forehead. This is due to the cleansing action of this practice on the sinuses and is nothing to worry about. Many experience clearer eyesight when practising this exercise. It is also very beneficial in centering and grounding us and bringing clarity to mind, body and spirit. Ideally practice daily for about 5—10 minutes.

BREATHING EXERCISE 3

ALTERNATIVE NOSTRIL BREATHING - (WITHOUT RETENTION)

This practice is best suited to those who prefer a simplified breathing practice. In this practice it is more or less the same as the previous breathe accept there is no retention/no holding of the breath.

It goes as follows;

- Block off left nostril (Starting point);
- Inhaling through right nostril (1);
- Block of right nostril (2);
- Exhale through left nostril (3);
- Inhaling left (then block nostril);
- Exhaling right;
- Inhaling right (then block nostril);
- Exhaling left;
- Inhaling left (then block nostril);
- Exhale right;

Do 5 rounds to start with as above.

The benefits of this practice are the same as the previous exercise. This practice has a great cooling affect on the head/forehead and mind. It is great for clearing up blocked sinuses and infection.

Take a few moments after practice to notice how the body feels, noticing, feeling and sensing what is going on. Those who practice Yoga will know the feeling of relaxation that comes over the body. The body remembers how it feels and you will want to do it again and again and again! Such bliss!

SECTION 7
INTERNAL FOCUS

After meditation, relaxation and visualisation it is important to know how you felt before, during and after the practice. For many of us the benefits of the practice go on hours after we have finished and it is important that we remember this and can feel the benefits. Why, well we'll come back and do it again. Our body will be very grateful for it. Notice how your body feels from focusing on the breath alone, nothing else to focus on just the breath and how this gentle exercise has brought about a kind of inner peace, harmony, inner glow. Taping this exercise is a good idea until you become familiar with it but it is not too difficult to understand. If you only ever learn one breathing technique this one is marvellous for just shutting down the monkey brain! The endless chitchat that goes on in our minds.

The beauty of meditation is that it is so simple and it doesn't cost you anything. The simplicity of it is what I love and the fact that we can perform it any time we choose. There are of course many different types of meditation out there but I tend to use the simplest forms. The ones that utilise the breath. The ones that don't take a great deal of thought, as, after all, the whole aim of meditation is to stop the brain from overworking, giving it a rest, a break from its daily routine. Often when we feel stressed the best thing to do is to sit in a quiet space, dark if you wish and just sit. Closing your eyes and just listening to the breath. This is basic meditation.

This internal focus, the watching and listening to the breath give us so much benefit. This moment of tranquillity, the slowing down of the mind is such a tonic to our whole system. Society today thrives on stress that is why there are so many heart attacks and illness and people dying at such a young age. The secret is to take this time out. If you can make 10 minutes each evening to just lie down or sit, which ever you prefer and listen to your breathing, internal awareness. You can even sit and picture you organs, from the head down to the feet, including all the internal organs. Something like this:

Sitting comfortable or lying down whichever you prefer, gently close your eyes, not tight, just gentle so the eyelids touch, allow your body to relax (against the floor) or allowing the shoulders to release and relax (if sitting), now slowly take the awareness to just outside the tip of your left nostril and notice the air as you breathe in through the nostrils, its slightly cool, now as you exhale notice the air is warmer as it has entered your body and is now released on the exhalation. Continue with this process for a few more breaths, breathing in, cool air, breathing out, warmer, natural breathe, don't harness it, let it happen natural.

Now you are feeling relaxed, take your awareness into the body now, we are going on an internal journey so you can visit each place within you.

Our first stop is inside the nostrils, we breathe in now and we follow that breathe, that energy deep inside the nasal passage, it now works its way past down the throat, past the chest and into the lungs, picture the lungs, healthy, pink, strong and vibrant, filling up with fresh, clean energy as you breathe in, feel them expanding with the inhalation, now as you exhale, they empty and shrink as they push out all the stagnant energy, and you breathe in again, filling them up with pure energy, they expand, now leave the lungs, and as you continue to breathe naturally we will continue on our internal journey, moving gently and slowly from one organ to the next, gentle awareness of each and every muscles, cell and tissue.

We notice something pulsating behind our lungs, it's a beautiful colour, fresh and vibrant, beating in time with our breathe, it feels so released, it is our heart, the heart centre. We notice the magnificent organ that beats within us, always beating, always pumping, always healthy. We notice the muscles and tissues that surround our heart, how they support it and how they have no tension and release with each exhalation, softening and supporting but no tension. Releasing negativity and pain with each exhalation, as we inhale we feel the strong beating of the heart, its natural function, working to pump our blood around our body, working strongly, but with ease and such comfort, we love this place, its our heart of emotion and we feel very peaceful in this place.

We notice the cage that supports and protects these upper organs, the ribs. We notice how strong they are but also how soft they are, no tension, just supporting and protecting, soft, no stress, opening and expanding with the inhalation, allowing the lungs to fill and these organs to expand and work in unison, uniting our body with our breathe, a wonderful feeling just to know.

We move now to the liver, it's a magnificent colour, it to is working strongly, filtering our body, purifying our blood, its healthy and strong. We notice how it works with all the other organs in unison, our body pumping, beating, filtering, sifting, moving, relaxing, it's such a wonderful thing to know.

We move down past the lungs now, and we notice the diaphragm, we notice its movement as we breathe in and we breathe out, it moves on its own with no help from us, it is healthy and functioning perfectly.

We notice our intestines, our complex digestive system, the organs entwined, functioning with perfection, no tension here, our abdomen softens as we exhale, the natural rhythm of the body moving and assisting our intestines to process and digest and eliminating toxins from our body. These large organs, entwined, working together, feeling relaxed and comfortable, as they support our system in many ways.

Moving down now to the reproductive organs, the pink fresh, vibrant area below. The most feminine part of us. This area thriving and pumping with fresh energy, fresh blood, all stagnant energy being released with every exhalation. This whole area is energised and functioning perfectly. There is no tension here, just natural body rhythms, natural energies as a feeling of relaxation washes each and every organ. The ovaries seated naturally in their chosen place, rested and peaceful, the bladder, working hard but there is no tension in this organ, notice how each and every part of you in this area, bladder, uterus, fallopian tubes, ovaries, how they work together and feel energised and natural.

We visit the hip and groin area, we notice how these muscles inter-react with one another, supporting and protecting and we notice as we exhale how the tension releases from the hips and their sockets, how the muscles around these bones release and relax as we exhale. As we inhale we notice how energised this whole area feels. Hold onto this energy for a while; keep it in as it washes over the deepest parts of you. We move down to the legs and the knees and the feet and the toes, the soles of the feet, and we work our way back up the back of the body now, back of the legs, back of the knees, back of the thighs, to the base of the spine, seated deeply inside us at the base of our being.

Picture the base of the spine, how its sits comfortably, how it holds no tension even though it supports our frame, strong and energised muscles and tissues surround this part of us, keeping it safe and supported. We move our awareness all the way up the spine now, noticing each disc, each vertebrae and knowing that they all work and function together, naturally and gently, supporting our frame, each disc supported by strong muscles and fibres, each muscle working strong and perfectly. There is no tension in any area of our spine.

If you feel tension stay in this place for a while, breathing in to that area, and imagining the tension releasing with each exhalation. We notice the blood pumping around each part of our spine, energising each muscle, cell and bone, keeping them strong and active, as they to work in unison. Supporting our body in many ways.

We notice the network of nerves that are all over our body, from the top of the head to the tips of the toes, each nerve serving a purpose, working together. We notice the nerves that run down each leg to the tips of the toes, and we notice how smooth they feel, how perfect they function, no tension. We move down to the feet, moving now back up the sides of the legs, the thighs, the hips, the sides of the torso, upper torso, the outside of the chest, the armpit, the arms, the shoulders, the colour bones, the neck, the jaw, the ears, the sides of the face, the temples, the forehead, the top of the head and we bathe now in the beauty and tranquillity of knowing that we have visited our internal self, noticing the many functions that our body does even when we are asleep, carrying out these functions without our assistance, such a wonderful, natural process.

Our breath is natural and gentle and very calm. It seems to happen so natural that we almost forgot all about it as we went on this journey. Relaxing and releasing both our body and mind. Everything now functioning perfectly, no tension. This is your inner journey. You can come back to this place any time you like, connecting with yourself, noticing, focussing and releasing. If you have a particular place that needs some attention stay in that place for a while, picturing the organ functioning perfectly, releasing any negativity or tension felt in that area. Stay in that place until you feel ready to move onto the next.

This can be as long or short a journey as you like. It is up to you how long you want to spend inside! As I mentioned if you have a particular area you wish to focus on then remain there until you feel that the organ, muscle or area feels fine and you can move on to the next. You will feel many benefits from this practice. It will become second nature after a few practices. It is best to allow yourself a few minutes when you feel you have completed the journey. Don't just rush up and stand up. Open your eyes gently and become familiar with your surroundings. We can often go into quite a deep state with this inner journey. So take time to bring your body round after practising. Again use the breathe as a tool to bring yourself round. Deepen the breath and awaken the body gentle, bringing yourself back to the present moment.

This time out from everyday life, as you switch off the mind helps with Endo as it relaxes you. Anything that relaxes the mind will help you to cope better. It really will. When you practice any visualisation you can adapt it to how you wish. If you find one way works better for you, a simpler way, then use that method. It doesn't have to be about remembering colours, rituals etc. I have found meditation and visualisation in their simplest form have helped me. I find I cannot remember too much, it fogs my head but the simplest meditations and visualisations help me to switch off. They will give you many benefits. If you do find yourself nodding off, then so be it, it is, as I have mentioned before, the time your body needs to rest, heal and relax.

I cannot stress enough how important and vital this 'switching off' and relaxing time is. Especially when we switch off the chitchat. The most beautiful thing about meditation and any relaxation technique is that your subconscious mind will remember how you feel and you will want to come back to that moment, practising time and time again, relaxing and releasing the mind and in turn that will release your body. If you only take one thing away from this book, take the meditations, the visualisations and the advice to switch off. Its vital and necessary for the society that we live in today.

SECTION 8
YOGA NIDRA—(Rotation of Consciousness)

Here is a routine called ***YOGA NIDRA*** which I mentioned briefly earlier. This practice involves the Corpse pose and is very beneficial for the whole body. The aim is to focus on different parts of the body and move from part to part, allowing the mind to only focus on certain body parts, thus allowing the rest of the mind to relax and switching off the monkey brain. (*You might like to tape the section in italics*). This practice is quite similar to the Inner Journey mentioned earlier. It involves bringing awareness briefly to certain areas of the body from the top to the bottom and moving round in a kind of synchronized fashion.

Here goes:

Lie in Corpse Pose. Keeping the eyes closed, simply listen to this tape and mentally follow these instructions. Do not move any part of the body; just take your awareness to it. Try not to lose consciousness or fall asleep.

Now focus on any external sounds. Moving your mind like a witness from one sound to another until it loses interest and becomes quite. This is ***'Antar Mouna'.***

Antar Mouna:

"When the mind is silent and peaceful it becomes very powerful. It can become a receptor of bliss and wisdom enabling life to become a spontaneous flow and expression of joy and harmony. However…this inner silence cannot arise while there is a continual stream of disturbing thoughts and emotions. All this inner noise of thoughts and emotions has to be removed before one can truly experience the soundless sound of inner silence". - ***Swami Satyananda Saraswati***

In this peaceful state is now the time to make your resolve, your '**Sankalpa**'. Choose a goal that is important to you and stick to that same resolve until the goal is reached or your needs change. Use clear, positive language to penetrate your unconscious mind. Where the resolve works like a seed planted in fertile soil.

Sankalpa:

A Sanskrit word meaning will; purpose; determination." A solemn vow or declaration of purpose to perform any ritual observance. Most commonly, sankalpa names the mental and verbal preparation made by a temple priest as he begins rites of worship. So Sankalpa will be your own personal purpose statement, I will be more understanding, I will be a pure vessel for healing, I will be etc, anything you wish but you have to see it through. It's your kind of promise to the Universe.

You can begin your resolve "from this moment on I am becoming more and more…" or "from this moment on I will be more. (Insert anything you choose). This will indicate that the desired change is happening from this moment on now for the unconscious mind lives in the present and tomorrow never comes.

Now we will begin the ***Rotation of Consciousness:***

We will now take your mind around your body. You are just to bring awareness to that part of you and not move it.

On your next inhalation please bring your awareness to:

- *Your right hand*
- *Your right thumb*
- *Your first finger*
- *Second finger*
- *Third finger*
- *Fourth finger*
- *Your right wrist*
- *Forearm*
- *Elbow*
- *Upper arm*
- *Shoulder*
- *Armpit*
- *Right side*
- *Waist*
- *Right hip*
- *Front of the right thigh*
- *Back of the thigh*
- *Right knee*
- *Back of the knee*
- *Calf*
- *Back of the calf*
- *Shin*
- *Ankle*
- *Heel*
- *Sole of foot*
- *Instep*
- *Top of foot*
- *Big toe*
- *Second toe*
- *Third toe*
- *Fourth toe*
- *Fifth toe, little toe*
- *Left hand*
- *Thumb*
- *First finger*
- *Second finger*
- *Third finger*
- *Fourth finger*
- *Left wrist*
- *Forearm*
- *Elbows*
- *Upper left arm*

- *Shoulder*
- *Armpit*
- *Left side*
- *Waist*
- *Left hip*
- *Front of thigh*
- *Back of thigh*
- *Knee*
- *Back of left knee*
- *Calf*
- *Shin*
- *Ankle*
- *Heel*
- *Sole of foot*
- *Instep*
- *Top of foot*
- *Big toe*
- *Second toe*
- *Third toe*
- *Fourth toe*
- *Fifth toe*
- *(Pause for 5 seconds)*
- *Now bring your awareness to your forehead*
- *Right eye*
- *Left eye*
- *Right temple*
- *Left temple*
- *Right ear*
- *Left ear*
- *Right cheek*
- *Left cheek*
- *Right nostril*
- *Left nostril*
- *Upper lip*
- *Lower lip*
- *Fell the tongue resting on the palate*
- *Feel the point of contact of both lips*
- *Chin*
- *Throat*
- *Right collarbone*
- *Left collarbone*
- *Right side of chest*
- *Left side of chest*
- *Right side of abdomen*
- *Left side of abdomen*
- *Waist*

- *Front of left leg*
- *Front of right leg*
- *Both legs together*
- *Groin*
- *Abdomen*
- *Belly button*
- *Chest*
- *Rib cage*
- *Centre of chest (sternum)*
- *Feel the movement of the chest as the breath moves in and out*
- *Neck*
- *Face*
- *Layers of skin on the face*
- *Forehead*
- *Top of head*
- *Back of head*
- *Neck*
- *Upper back*
- *Right shoulder blade*
- *Left shoulder blade*
- *Right arm and hand*
- *Left arm and hand*
- *Right side of back*
- *Left side of back*
- *Spine*
- *Lower back*
- *Right buttock*
- *Left buttock*
- *Back of right leg/heel*
- *Back of left leg/heel*
- *Back of both legs*
- *Buttocks*
- *Lower back*
- *Upper back*
- *Back of head*
- *Top of head*
- *Forehead*
- *Right eye*
- *Left eye*
- *Right nostril*
- *Left nostril*

Awareness of the breath in the nasal passage. Now watch your breathing, watch the navel rise and fall with the breath. Count the naval breaths backwards from 30 down to 1, starting again if you make a mistake.

Now watch the chest moving with the breath and count the chest breaths from 20 down to 1.

Now watch the breathe in the nostril and count the nostril breaths from 20 down to 1.

Remember your resolve and repeat it "from this moment on I will be.... plant the see that will begin to grow from this moment on.

Now very gently bring your awareness back to the room. Feel your back against the mat, feel your body lying against the floor, feel the breath as it enters the nostrils as you inhale, and as you exhale. Become familiar with your surroundings. Deepen the breath and begin to wake the body up. When you are ready roll over to your right side before coming into a seated position.

When seated:

Bring your hands in front of you and rub them vigorously. Rubbing your thighs and arms, now rubbing the hands again, and place them over your eyes, close the eyes, breathing in the energy from the hands; now taking the hands down in prayer position, forehead to the floor, Namaste. This completes the practice. Remember how your body feels now after this session.

SECTION 9
Chakras (Our Energy Centres)

Believe it or not our bodies have many energy centres located at different parts of the body. In Yogic terms these spinning discs of energy are called "Chakras". There are many thousands of them located inside of our bodies, but we are only going to concentrate on the 7 main ones. It has not been proven that the Chakras exist because to modern man he needs proof, something tangible that he can prod and touch and say "well, yes I guess that's a Chakra" but the Chakras do exist, although they are not tangible but they are an important part of us as human beings and we can learn to understand them and use them to keep us healthy. I am only going to touch on these lightly and show you a few basic visualisation techniques and meditation techniques that help to calm your mind and de-stress you.

It can be as simple as just lying down and taking your awareness to the parts of the body that each Chakra is related to. I mentioned earlier at the beginning of the book that it is in this quiet time of no thinking, no sleeping, just being that we can truly be ourselves and our bodies can begin to take a breather and heal. Don't be afraid to try the exercises. You are fully in control every step of the way and as I have so often said to my Yoga students, if you fall asleep then so be it, your body obviously needed to rest. There are 7 main Chakras. They are located along the spinal column at specific areas as outlined below. I shall touch briefly on their purpose.

The first is the base or root Chakra or ***Muladhara Chakra*** as it is called in Sanskrit. It is located below the sacrum bone at the perineum or the base of the spine. The colour here is red. This Chakra is concerned with our inner wisdom. Call it our survival Chakra, grounding us, what we are, our purpose etc. A child's root Chakra is ever pure, balanced and in harmony as they have not yet experienced life and are non-judgemental. As we grow older and experience life, many experiences unbalance and affect us which in turn affects our root Chakra, root centre. To bring this back in balance has a profound affect on our entire system. We know who we are, know where we are going etc, and nothing concerns us, we are at one. It is basically a very grounding Chakra. Reuniting us with positivity and purpose.

The second Chakra is located just up from the root Chakra and is known as the Sacral Chakra, or ***Swadhisthana***. Its associated colour is orange and it is located just behind the belly button. This is the creativity Chakra. Our centre of attention and knowledge. Physically it is connected with our Liver, Kidneys and lower stomach/abdomen. When over utilised, that is we think too much this centre becomes drained of vital energy and illness such as Diabetes or Cancer can occur only when this centre is completely out of balance.

The third is ***Manipura*** Chakra; a sunny, golden Chakra, its colour is yellow or golden like the sun, it is located just a few inches up from the second Chakra and is located in the stomach area or solar plexus. This is associated with courage, satisfaction and contentment with life and all that that surrounds us.

The fourth Chakra is located at the heart centre and its name is ***Anaharta*** Chakra. The associated colour here is green or pink like that of a Rose. This Chakra is concerned with our feelings, love and happiness, true love of the self, our spirit and soul. Often this Chakra is blocked if we don't feel loved and therefore are incapable of giving out love. If out of balance this Chakra can cause symptoms such as Asthma, various lung and heart conditions. It is this centre, which deals with how we act and respond to others. Letting love into our hearts makes the journey easier. It gives us a sense of well-being, giving of the self, not being selfish and often it is harder work to be angry, selfish etc. Being unselfish and allowing love to flow from the heart brings us many benefits. When working with this Chakra, to open it and balance it is wonderful. All doubts, fears etc vanish and become so unimportant. Things we may dwell on and hold inside are released and it is exactly that kind of feeling, a releasing and unburdening.

I find this Chakra one of the most important to work with, especially with Endo. You can visualise this Chakra as green like an emerald or pink like a rose. This helps us in a physical sense by opening up the heart centre when we visualise it and it can help ease chest complaints such as Asthma and Angina. If we learn to unlock the tension in our hearts then we can be truly free from emotional pain.

The fifth Chakra is called ***Vishudda*** and it is located at the top of the spine at the back of the throat. Its colour is blue, (remember it is your shade of the colours given. Don't concentrate too hard on a particular shade of blue; use the one that comes into your mind. It may take a while if you are not used to visualising. I find it helps if say you need to picture orange but can't, then bring into your minds eye an actual orange! Then picture it where that associated Chakra centre is). In time you will be able to go to that place that colour and know the name. It becomes second nature. Honest, and it does not take too long at all. When we concentrate and open this centre all guilt feeling and remorse vanish. We speak clearly, from the heart. We don't feel the need to *be heard* to have to shout to have our point heard, we feel at one.

The sixth Chakra is called ***Ajna*** and it is located between the eyebrows. Its associated colour is indigo or purple, whichever is easier for you to visualise. This is associated with insight and how we look at life from within. It is said that it is our third eye and can open us up to psychic potential if we work with it. Working with this centre we dissolve ego, self-centeredness. We open our inner mind, our insight to greater things. It releases false identity, misidentifications, things like imbedded ideals, racialism etc. It frees us and helps us to see a greater picture. It is a very releasing Chakra, very freeing. Almost opening up to the earth and all that is in it.

The final Chakra is called ***Sahrasrara*** - the crown Chakra, located at the very top of the head. The colours associated with this Chakra are gold, silvers or bright white light. Again it is up to you which colours you can visualise with ease. This is a wonderful centre and we can use this on its own to bring in fresh energy, golden or silver light whenever we feel down. It is our immediate opening to the universal energy that is available for us all and is in such abundance and it is free! This 7th Centre is an integration of the other 6th and works in harmony to balance our entire being. Often we have limited concepts, limited imagination, and limited perception.

This centre opens that up and there are endless limitations, there are no barriers, we are free. If you have never worked with the energy centres before you may be presently surprised at how you feel when you use them. There are many methods to use the Chakras for healing, de-stressing, meditation and relaxation. The key is that each and every one of us will see different shades of colour associated for our own unique individuality. Don't concentrate too hard and don't become frustrated. In time you will become familiar with the practice. It is enough just to focus on the colours. The opening and balancing will take care of itself with you just initiating the process! See simple! If you find it difficult to visualise certain colours or awareness of location then stay with that Chakra area until you feel comfortable. Again, in time it will be second nature and with the help of the Chakra Man image I have attached for you, you will know which area to work on. A weekly Chakra session really helps. Spending 20—30 minutes relaxing and focusing on the centres and becoming aware of them. This quiet time is really important and brings you and connects you to the inner you!

BASIC CHAKRA VISUALISATION

Lie down on the floor or on a mat, on your back. This posture is called the Corpse pose and is one of the hardest to do because it is in this posture that we learn to relax fully, to let go and unwind, no thought, no speech, no chat, just being. Creating that quiet time. Many people find this very hard to do as they cannot let go and relax fully. Escaping from this world for a few moments. It is in this quiet time our bodies can heal, unburden our mind and leave us feeling refreshed. If you only practice for 10 minutes it is not important. The important thing is that you have taken this special time for your self and your body will still benefit. Try and visualise the colours, see them in your third eye, Ajna, point behind the forehead. If you fall asleep so be it. Don't worry about it. Enjoy it, it just means you needed to rest that's all!

Let's Begin:

Finding your comfortable position, as you begin to relax against the floor, focus on the point of your nose just outside of the left nostril and begin to inhale, taking that breathe deep down to the abdomen, watching it rise. When you are ready to naturally exhale, exhale feeling the abdomen fall gently back down.

Repeat—inhaling, exhaling, inhaling exhaling for about 5 minutes, allowing your mind and body to relax.

When you are ready to begin, keeping the breathing natural, take your awareness to the root Chakra, located deep in the seated area, lower spine, try and picture the area as a red disk of energy spinning clockwise. Visualise this if you can, if you can't no worries, don't force it, just bringing your awareness to the root centre is enough. Feel it balancing as you remain there for a few moments, relaxing further with each exhalation. If you can visualise the colour and the spinning disk work to balance it and if it seems to be spinning too fast just slow it down, focusing, relaxing.

When you are ready to move to the next energy centre bring your awareness a little further up the spine to the sacral centre located just below the belly button. The colour here is orange, work on focusing, noticing, sensing this energy centre and if you can picture it spinning in a clockwise direction at a speed that feels comfortable to you then do so. It is enough to just focus and become aware of the colour spinning in a clockwise direction. If you experience difficulty with visualising the clockwise spinning just become aware of the colour in that part of the spine/body.

Remain here until you are ready to move to the next Chakra, the Solar Plexus, located in the stomach area, behind the belly button. The colour here is yellow, golden like the sun, work on the visualisation, spinning disk, or again if this is not for you just bringing your awareness to this area. Stay here until you are satisfied that the area is filling up with the colour and feels balanced. If it is difficult to focus on the colour stay with it until you can. Now we are ready to move to the Heart centre.

Moving up to behind the chest where your heart is located. Imagine a spinning disc of green energy, or imagine the chest lighting up with green as the heart expands and opens. Allow yourself to stay here for a few moments, visualising the balancing green energies. If you prefer you can use pink/rose colours to soften the heart centre. When you feel balanced then move to the next centre, located at the top of the spine at the back of the throat area.

This is the throat Chakra, its colour is blue. Stay with this colour and imagine the colour spinning, bright vibrant blue, clearing your throat and balancing the energies in this area. If you cannot visualise the spinning disk then just become aware of this area at the top of the spine, the back of the throat and the associated colour is blue. When you are ready move to the third eye centre.

This is located in between the eyebrows, behind the forehead. You can picture this indigo/violet whichever is easier. If you like just bring your awareness to this area and imagine it clearing, clear, cool and empty with no clutter, no chit chats. If you can imagine the colours then you can picture the spinning disk of energy, vibrant indigo/violet energy, cool, clear and cleansing. If you want to you can visualise a large eye in this area, like that of a Buddha. This will help to strengthen your insight or psychic ability. When you are ready, and feel balanced in this centre, move to the final Chakra.

Located at the very top of the head, this is the Crown centre. You can imagine it as a lotus flower with a thousand petals opening and enlightening. You can imagine this area opening and a bright golden or white/silver light entering the crown of your head and washing over your entire body, balancing your very soul, energising and revitalising. Imagining the energy of the sun entering every part of you, muscle, cell, and organ, rejuvenating and filling you with vibrant fresh new energy. Some can visualise themselves being taken up into the light and bathing in it as they lie there. This takes practice but go with what you feel comfortable with.

This is a very balancing practice and you can tape this practice and play it back. As you become familiar with the colours and location of the energy centres it will be easier for you to do this automatically. If you feel yourself nodding off don't worry. It just means that is what your body needs to do! As I mentioned briefly earlier if you find it difficult initially to visualise the spinning disk of energy it is enough to just focus on the area along the spine, the associated area of the body and just bring your awareness there until you feel balanced. With regular practice this will become easier for you.

The 'Chakra Man ©' image inserted below will assist you.

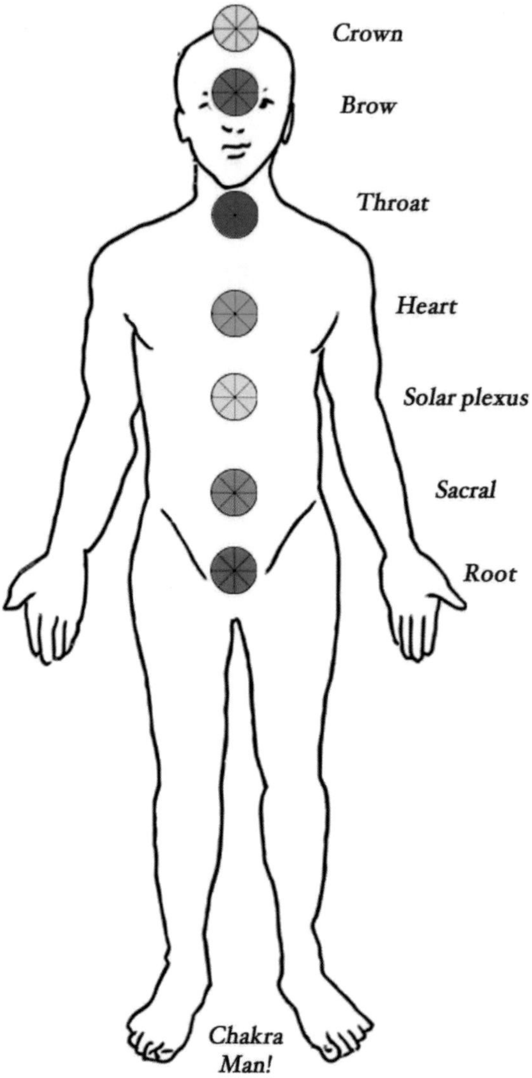

SECTION 10
YOGA

BEFORE WE BEGIN

As with anything new and unfamiliar it is important to be properly prepared. In Yoga there are certain postures that carry warnings or *contra-indications.* That is to say that some people who have certain health problems may not be able to do certain postures or should at least consult their GP beforehand. A good Yoga Practitioner will always ask you this before commencing class or practice.

The postures outlined in this book are basic beginner postures. They do not carry any contra-indications however, I would ask that if you do suffer from any of the following that you check with your GP beforehand that it is ok to practice. These are basic postures, designed for those with Endometriosis and are safe and simple to use.

- Angina
- Heart Illness
- Lung Illness (*Asthma is not included here*)
- Blood Clots
- Emphysema
- High Blood Pressure (*extreme cases)*
- Low Blood Pressure (*extreme cases)*
- Diabetes
- Severe back problems such as slipped or prolapsed disc.

The list above relates to *serious cases of the above.* Some Yoga postures are very beneficial for such things as low and high blood pressure but again it is always best to speak to your GP before practising. These postures, routines and breathing techniques are aimed at relaxing the body and purifying from the inside out. Calming the mind, releasing tension, de-stressing. As well as relaxing, the routines, especially *Sun* Salutes, wake up the whole body, working on all the systems within the body and give us a complete massage, inside and out. None of the postures are difficult.

Yoga is a beautiful journey. If you become more flexible then you can move on to more advanced Yoga postures and invest in DVDs, books etc. The postures outlined within these pages are designed for Endo sufferers; they are gentle and not too intense. Work slowly and remember the internal focus, don't just do it, feel it. Some postures like the Dog will mean that you are nearly upside down. Putting the body into some odd positions.

There is nothing to fear here. When the heart is lower than the head, as it is in *Dog posture* the heart gets a real good massage. People take up Yoga for many different reasons. I took it up as I immediately felt the benefits. These benefits have enhanced my life and health in so many ways. Don't be frightened to try new things. Work with your body and experience the stretches, the bends, relaxation and the de-stressing.

Don't just do the postures - feel them. Yoga has so many postures that can be used to target specific ailments and Illness within our bodies. There are postures to get rid of neck tension, headaches, backache, bloated and wind! They can all help in Endo pain relief. Tried and tested, trusted postures to bring that all important balance and harmony. The breathing practices are simple ones. I have learned from my own experience that watching my breathe, in a relaxed atmosphere, whether it is after a hot bath or just shutting the world out for a few minutes a day is what has helped me cope with Endo. You will need the following to practice (but don't go out and buy the most expensive) a decent yoga mat should cost around £12—16 pounds.

- Yoga Mat
- Blanket
- Belt or strap
- Pillow
- Yoga blocks or/and cushions

The yoga mat is used so that you don't slip when performing the postures (Asanas). The blanket is used after practice when doing relaxation in Corpse Pose. When we meditate our body temperature drops slightly. Belt or strap to use when stretching. This stops us overstretching and hurting ourselves. The belt can be your best friend and you work together and become more flexible. The pillow is needed for those of you who don't like to have your head flat on the floor and cushions/blocks can also be used for this. You can also use the pillow for underneath the lower back or under the knees, depending on whether you feel any discomfort whilst lying down. The blocks or cushions can be used to sit on especially when doing seated postures when opening up the hips, as they can help to release the hip and groin area.

It is best to practice Yoga at least 2 hours after eating. This gives the food time to digest and the body to settle. You don't want to be doing a headstand just after your tea. Many people are put off by Yoga initially. When they hear Yoga they immediately picture someone very supple with their legs behind their head and this is a shame because the people that can do that are very supple and have probably been practising Yoga for many years. I am not asking you to do that here.

The aim of this section is to introduce you to simple Yoga. Yoga that can balance and energise you from the inside out. Yoga should not be seen as a chore; it should not be an effort to get going. The beauty with Yoga is that you will feel the benefits straight away and with this daily routine you will soon be toning up from the inside out along with bringing that all important union of mind, body and spirit. In the simple postures and routines that will follow I am not asking you to tie your legs in a knot or chant OM at the top of your voice, of course we can go into that if you wish but these routines are simple and basic to use and remember and I have kept it simple.

By doing routines either first thing in the morning or early evening, before you retire (1—2 hours before sleeping) two or three times a week, or daily if you so wish, you will keep your body flexible, fit and supple. You do not have to be overly flexible this will come with regular practice. I don't do a complete Yoga session each day, some days I don't do anything but I know how I feel after doing gentle stretches, bends and twists and so I always come back to it. (Yoga Postures are called 'Asanas' but I will refer to them as postures).

The postures outlined are the basic postures that many of us learn when we are introduced to Yoga. You can perform these on their own or develop a routine, a flowing sequence of postures such as those included in Sun Salutes which we will cover later. Here are some basic postures, names and a brief outline of their benefits:

(Please note some postures should be avoided during menstruation. I will highlight the ones that you should avoid).

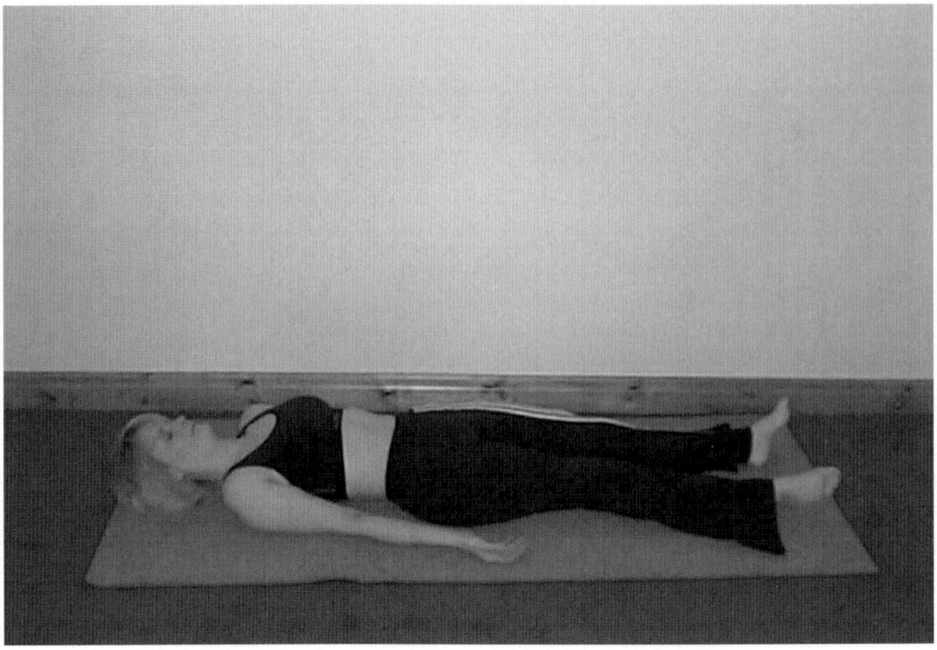

Corpse Pose

This posture is often done at the beginning of practice and at the end. It is actually quite hard to do, as the aim is to lie completely still and allow the body and mind to switch off.

<u>How it's done:</u>

- Lying down on your back on a mat. Now finding that comfortable position we work from the top of the head down:

- Take your chin gently forward towards the notch in the chest, this opens up the back of the head and neck area.

- Allow your back to release against the floor. If you have back pain you can bring your knees up and place your feet on the floor for comfort but ideally you just want to lie flat. A blanket can be placed under the back if necessary.

- Allow the feet to flop out to the sides; the arms should be about 3—5 inches away from the side of the body, palms facing up, and fingers passive. If the back feels tense, lift up the buttocks gently and move the torso forward, stretching gently from the waist down, placing the buttocks back on the floor.

- You can shuffle the legs down one by one if you wish to extend a little. The feet should be equal distance apart so take them about 30cm width apart and bring the big toes in to meet each other then take them apart again allowing them to flop out to the sides.

- In this posture there is no tension. You gently close the eyes, not tight, just gently, and take awareness to just outside the tip of the left nostril. To relax in the posture you use the breath. In through the nose, out through the nose, inhaling, exhaling. When you breathe in you breathe past the lungs and take the breath deep down to the abdomen. Something to note:

YOU NEED TO NOTICE HERE THE INHALATION—AND WHAT THE ABDMOMEN DOES. REMEMBER PROPER BREATHING LIKE A BABY. AS YOU INHALE THE ABDOMEN GENTLY EXPANDS, AS YOU EXHALE IT RELEASES BACK DOWN. THIS IS YOUR FOCUS.

INHALE—ABDOMEN RISES
EXHALE—ABDOMEN FALLS

If you breathe into the upper chest you are not taking a complete full breathe in. If you breathe in and the abdomen rises then you are taking a complete breath. This takes a little getting used to initially. To notice this even more until you become familiar with the breathing process it may help you to place the hands beside the Belly Button, left hand on left side, right hand on right side and fingertips of opposite hands touching just across where the belly button is. As you breathe in the fingertips come apart ever so slightly as the abdomen expands. As you exhale the fingertips touch again, come back together on the exhalation. You may like to repeat this for a few breaths so you become used to the process.

So the aim of Corpse pose is to:

- *Get in the comfortable position;*
- *Allowing the body to relax against the floor;*
- *Using the breath to relax further, with every exhalation your body sinks further into the floor;*
- *No tension, no stress just being...lying on the floor, breathing, no movement;*
- *Creating that quiet, tranquil moment where there is no thought. Focusing only on the breath and the pattern of it, the movement of the abdomen. This is how we switch off.*

In the initial stages you may find you nod off! That's perfectly acceptable. You can use this pose to relax the mind and body, to calm yourself after a long day in the office, to get in tune with yourself when the outside world gets a little hectic. You can use it before practice to centre and align the body and rest the mind. You then use it to end a Yoga session so that your body has time to relax and enjoy the benefits of practice. It is a wonderful posture on its own.

WARM UPS

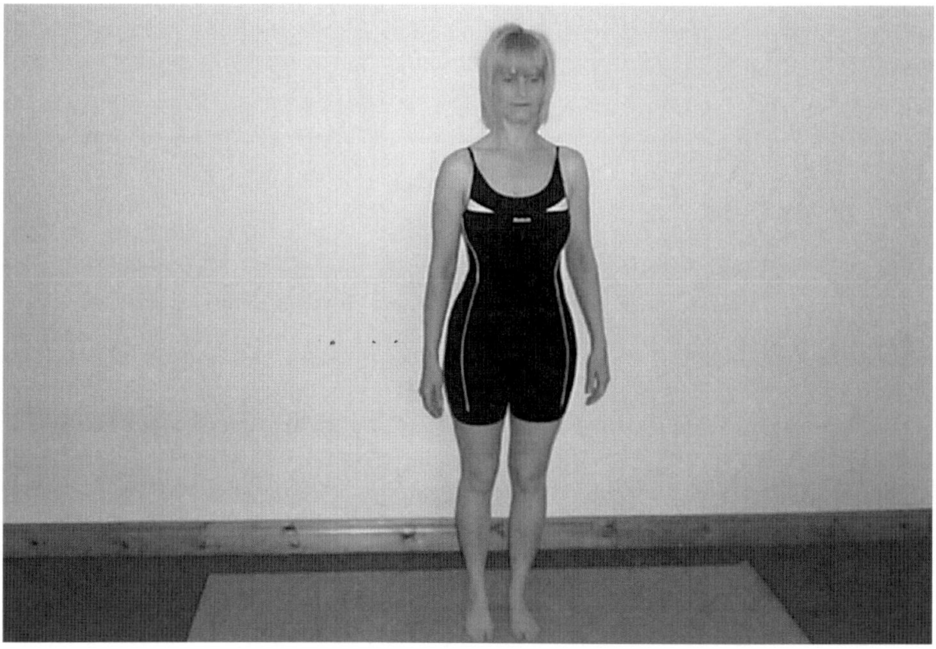

Mountain Pose / Standing Tall

It is vital that you warm up before practising as this prepares the body for posture work. Never rush into a workout or posture routine before warming up as you could injure yourself and that can lead to possible pain and discomfort. Warm ups do just that, they warm up the body, limbering and stretching so you are ready to practice. Here are a few sample warm-ups.

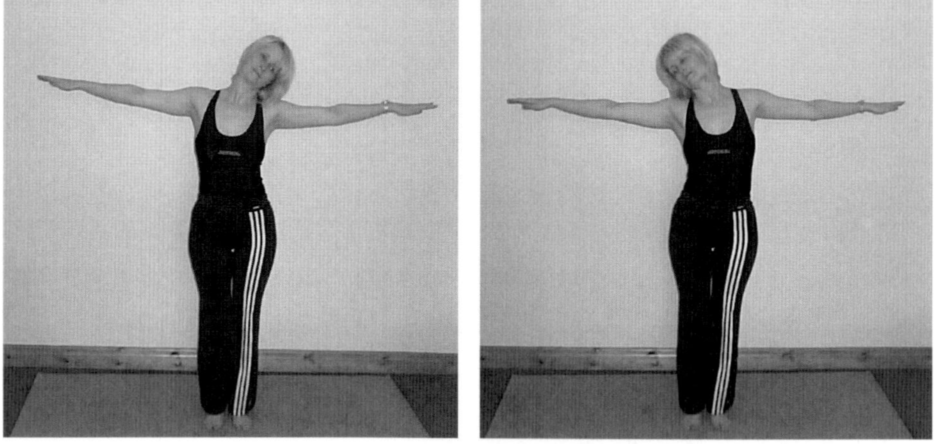

Gentle Neck Opening Exercise

- Standing tall, gently bring the left ear towards the left shoulder, not all the way but if you can great! If not just work on opening and stretching the neck, very gently.
- Then do same with opposite, right ear to right shoulder. Repeat 3 each side.

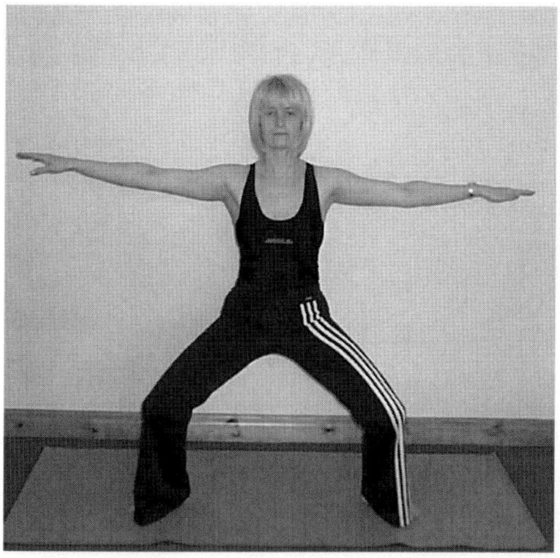
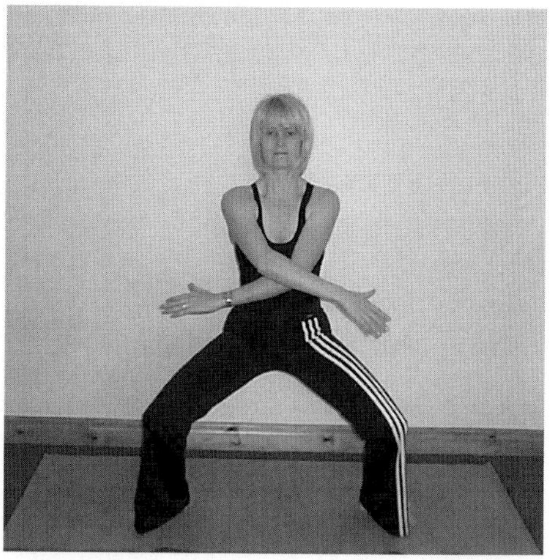

Windmill Stance

- (This is a strong posture and builds up stamina!).Standing tall, place the feet about 3 to 4 feet apart, the feet facing out at a 45° angle. then bend the knees, the feet should be pointed out away from the body.
- Your thighs should be parallel to the floor, and keep them strong, imagine them being like a tabletop.
- Find your balance and then dip the buttocks, drop them so you are kind of seated on an imaginary chair, drop the shoulders and take the arms wide, inhaling get ready.
- Slowly begin to rotate the arms crossing left over right in front of you, in big circles so they cross at the front of the body, do 10 circles clockwise then change and do 10 anti-clockwise.
- Keep the buttocks working strong and the legs. Great invigorating warm up.
- Keep the breath working with the posture, inhaling as the arms go up, exhaling as they come down. Rest at the end for a few breaths. The photos will help you to get into stance.

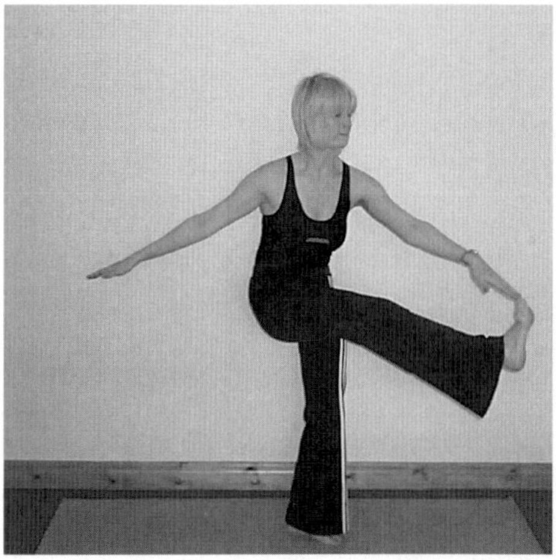 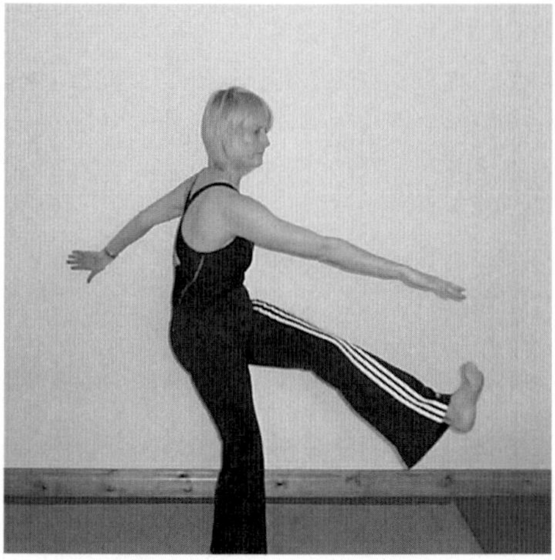

Leg / Arm Rotations

- Standing tall take the weight onto the left leg.
- Pressurise the left foot into the floor, this is grounding you.
- Inhale and at the same time raise the right leg straight up in front of you and try to touch your toes with your left hand. This is a balancing pose so take it slowly.
- When you have done one side, switch legs so the right leg becomes grounded, taking the weight and bring the left leg up, bringing the right hand to touch the left toes. As you develop and become stronger and more balanced, rotate your arms over your shoulders, behind, in big circular motions (see photo) and bring to your toe.
- Repeat on each side, left then right. Do for 3 reps each side.
- Exhaling as you reach for toes.
- Inhaling as you swap arms and take arm back to bring forward
- Repeat this 10 times, 5 each side in quick rotation.
- Rest at the end.
- Now standing tall, slight variation this time—do the process backwards, that is taking the left leg and bending the knee,
- Take it backwards and touch the sole of the left foot with right hand, release leg to floor and then take right leg, bend it behind and touch the right sole of foot with the left hand.
- Repeat and do quite fast changing leg and hand, do about 10 each side.
- Rest at the end, standing tall.

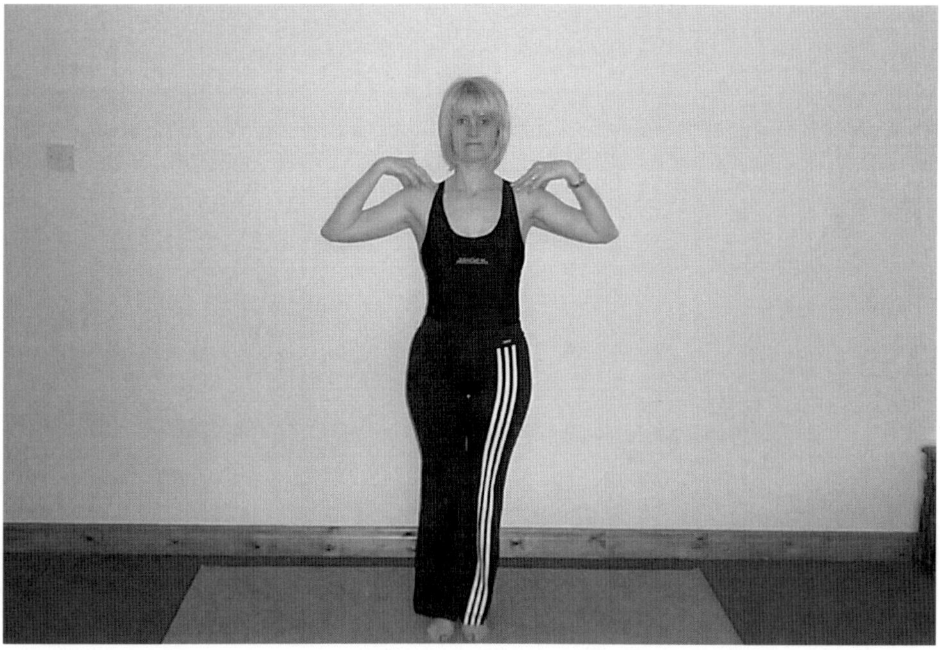

Arm Rotations

- Standing tall, place feet hip width apart,
- Now extend the arms out to the side, not too high,
- Touching the shoulders with the hands begin to rotate the arms clockwise 5 times and anti-clockwise 5 times,
- Then repeat same. Starting with little circles then working towards bigger circles, clockwise and then anti-clockwise.

This exercise works to free up the shoulders and eases pain from calcifications that can occur in the shoulders. It also helps to loosen upper back and the whole of the shoulders and arms.

Rest at the end bringing arms down and standing tall.

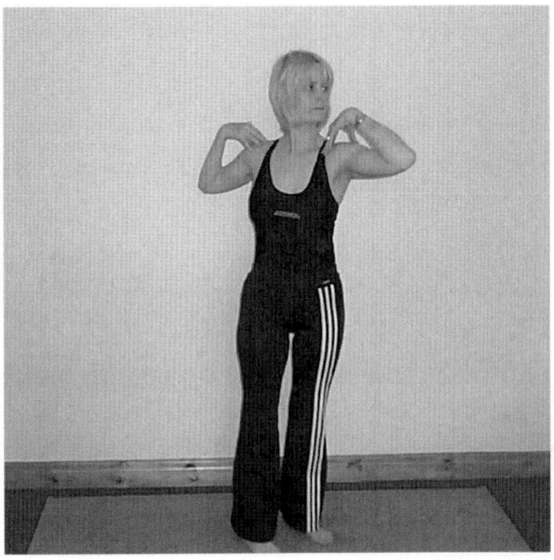 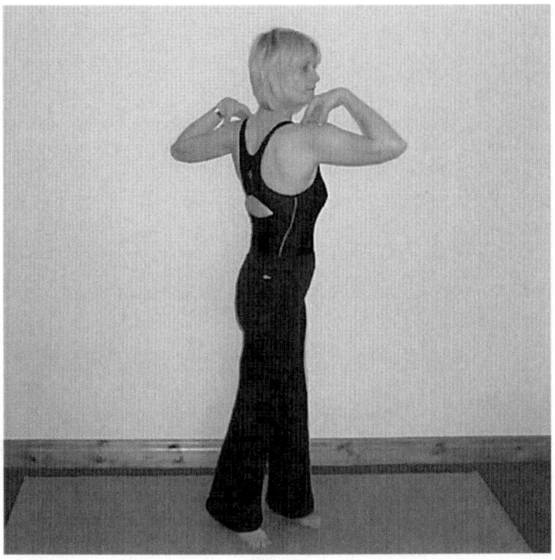

Torso Twists

- Standing tall feet facing forward and hip width apart,
- Place hands on shoulders, with elbows pointing out to the sides.
- Keeping the lower body facing forward, bring the right elbow pointing to the front, this moves the right elbow behind as you twist, don't move the lower body, just the waist and torso as you move left to right.
- Taking both arms towards the left, hold for a few seconds, inhale when turning, when turned exhale and soften into the pose, trying to twist further as you exhale, now turn back to centre then to opposite side.
- You should be working on keeping the lower body facing forwards throughout the practice and just moving the upper torso.
- Work with the breathe, this is the key to stretching and releasing, softening and toning the body. This pose is excellent not only as a warm up but for toning the waist and stomach/abs.

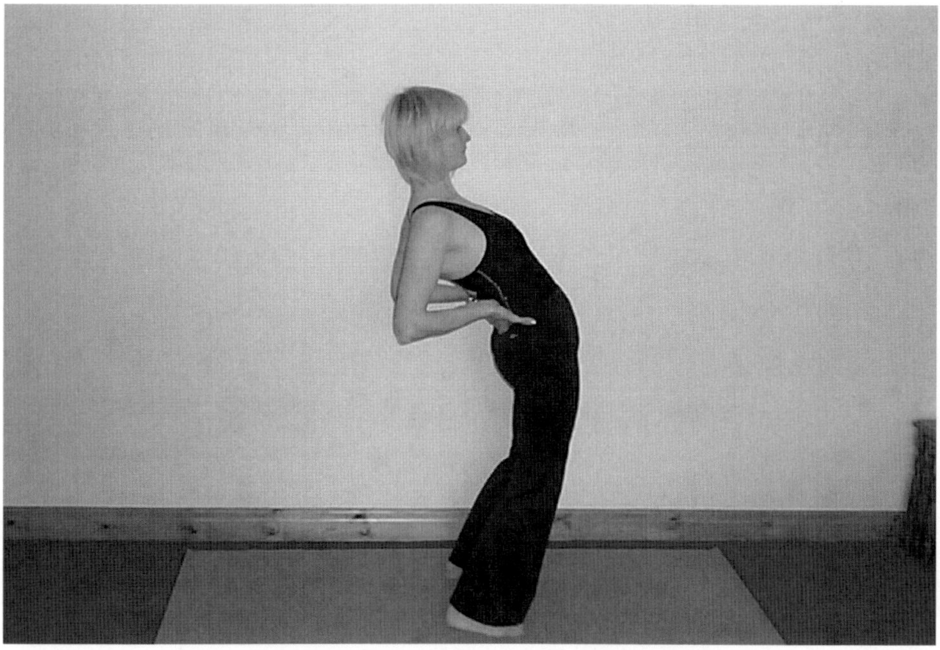

Back Arch / Opening Up Chest

- Standing tall, place the hands to the middle of the back,
- Inhale and when ready to exhale, lean back gently,
- Lift the head slightly but not right back.
- Feel the chest opening, pressurise the hands into the back slightly to open the chest and lean back a little further. Breathing naturally.
- Come back up slowly remaining in the pose for 5—10 seconds, enjoying the stretch.
- Then come up to standing, exhale and begin to roll the body forward, hands down by side, head and neck light as you take the body in the opposite direction, feeling the lower back stretching, lengthening and opening. Stay for about 10 seconds and then breathing in, roll back up gently to centre and then go backwards again as above.

Repeat this cycle 4 times:

- Back
- Centre
- Forward
- Centre
- (1 cycle)

This is another great warm up, opening the chest, working the arms, lengthening the spine ready for practice. Make sure your legs are strong and feet firmly on the floor.

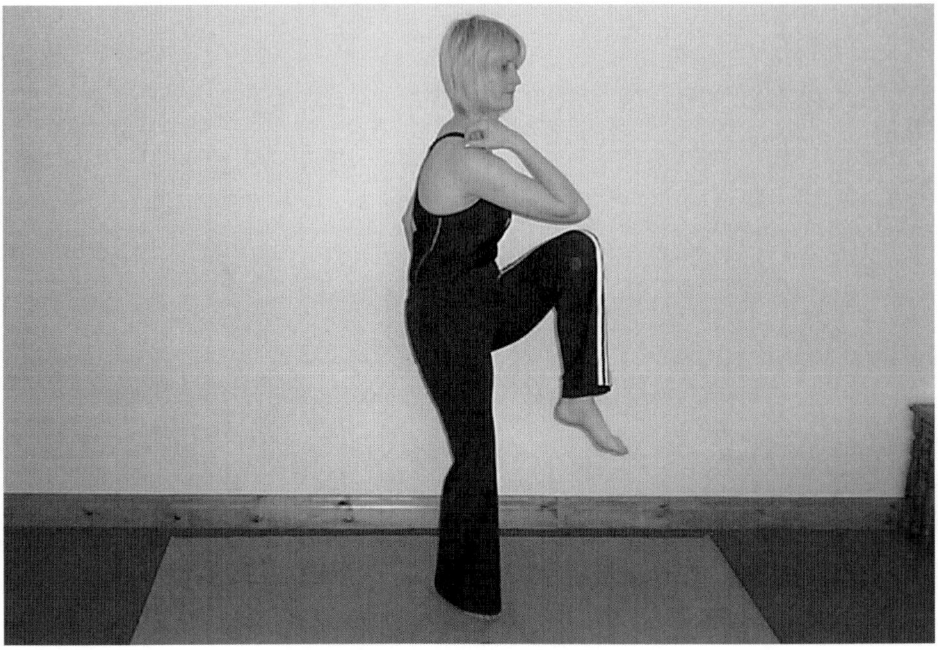

Knee to Elbow Routine

- Standing tall gently lift up the left leg, bending knee gently, and take the left elbow to knee.
- Release and work opposite side, right elbow to right leg.
- Do 5 of these.
- Now work opposites, that is lift up right leg and take left elbow to right knee, so you are crossing over the arm to knee.
- Work opposite side and do 5 reps.

This posture is great for co-ordination, balance and posture.

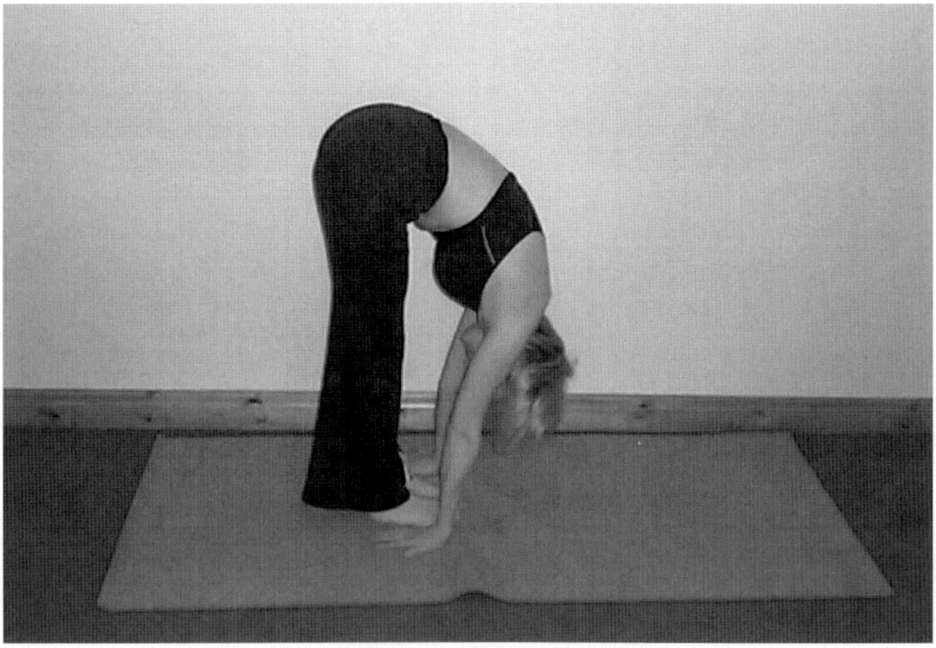

Forward Side Stretch

A great warm up to finish on:

- Standing tall, hands on hips, feet hip width apart, just allow the body to flop forward, and just hang, letting the back release, head and neck light, just hang there. (go into this posture controlled, don't rush it).
- Legs are strong; again legs are the foundation in this pose.
- Exhaling and lengthening. Remain for 30—60 seconds then come up on the inhalation arms out by sides and take a few breaths, exhaling and release back down one more time.

Remember to allow the head and neck to be light, no tension, just hang there. Come up on the inhalation to finish.

In the image above you will see my hands are right against the floor, this is an advanced version and takes time, just hanging there, with your legs strong, and the top of your body just hanging between your legs is fine. The head and upper body will release as you use the breath, the exhalation to lengthen further, don't rush it, it will come with time and the legs and hamstrings will release. It doesn't matter at what level of flexibility you are, just feel the posture, work on lengthening and opening up the back, keeping the legs firm on the ground as the legs and feet are the foundation to keep you firm. If you interlock the arms whilst bending forward the head will help the back release forward, like a weight. Always come out in a gentle, slow, and controlled fashion, never rush.

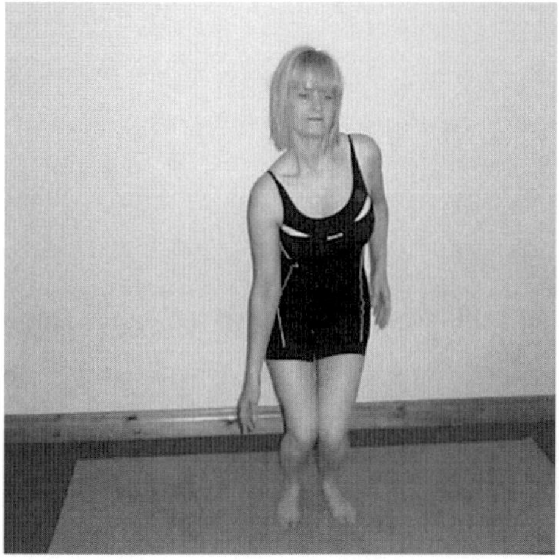

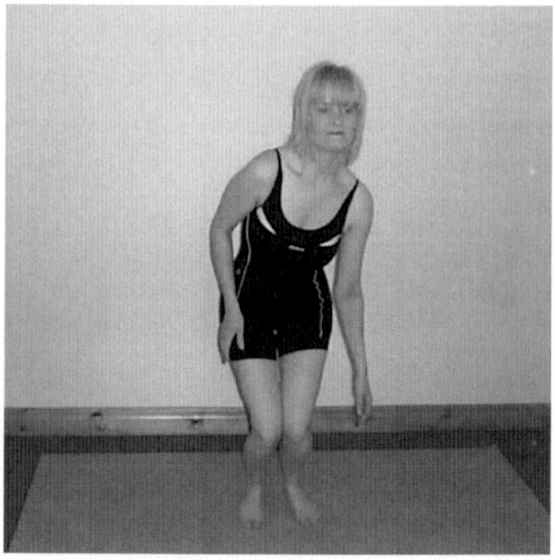

Body Shakes (Invigorating!)

- Stand tall and shake the arms from top of arm to fingers shake shake shake!
- Then lift left leg off floor, rotate ankles, clockwise, and anti-clockwise, then lift right leg and do same.
- Then stand tall and wriggle the body, shaking and wriggling as you bend the knees and work towards the floor and wriggle back up to standing. Very invigorating!

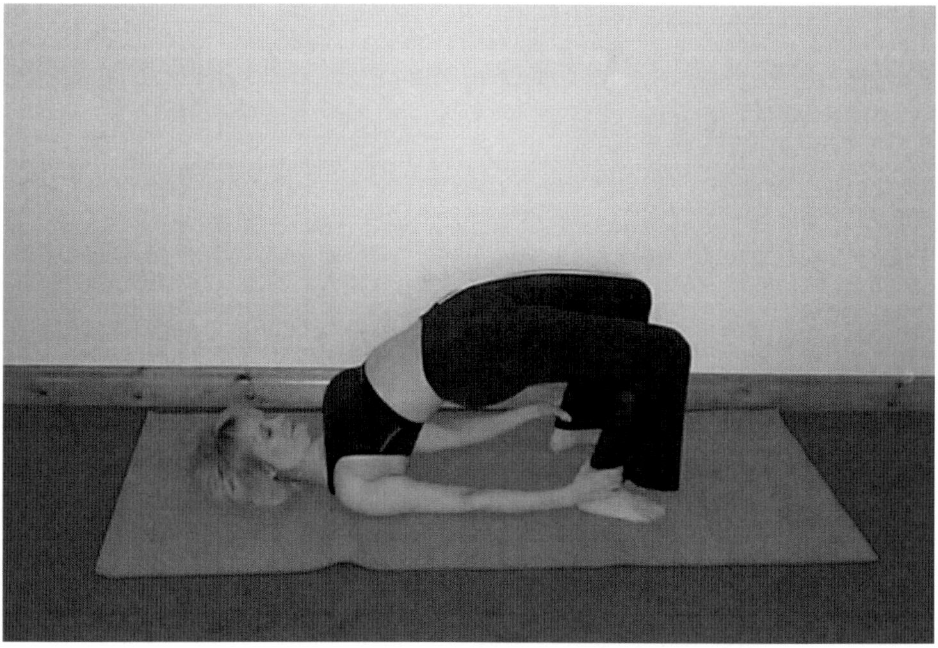

Bridge Pose - Avoid during Menstruation

The Bridge is a very strong posture. It works mainly on the back and helps to open the discs. It is also very beneficial for thyroid problems as the positioning of the neck in the full posture helps to massage the thyroid gland, bringing fresh energy and blood supply, releasing toxins and stagnant energy in this area. It is very beneficial for lower back problems and releases tension in the upper back and shoulders.

- Lying down flat on the floor bending the knees and bring your ankles as near to the buttocks as you can, keeping your feet flat on the mat. You can take hold of the ankles if you wish or the hands can be placed palm side down along the sides of the body.

- With the knees now bent, arms outstretched and palms flat against the floor, or holding the ankles (whichever you have chosen), using the feet push up from the floor, tensing the buttocks and keeping the thighs parallel to the floor. Keep the feet flat against the floor, this is your support. Using the feet to push against the floor helps you to maintain this posture.

You will notice the neck now comes into the chest as you push up the buttocks, the chest opens fully and the back arches over, get the feeling of pushing the hips up into the ceiling, opening up this area, buttocks tight. Try and focus on the abdomen, watching the stomach rising and falling. In this posture to begin with the breath may be rapid, deeper, try and control it.

The key to **Yoga Postures** is the use of the ***breathe*** within the posture so with BRIDGE posture the closing of the neck into the chest, the chest opening and the pushing of the legs and tensing of the buttocks all works on the breathe so it needs to be deep and controlled. It will be faster than usual but this is nothing to be concerned with. It is your body working hard in the posture.

- Try and keep the buttocks pushing up. The back arches and the hips push up. The feet strong, pushing into the floor. The breath easier as you work with the posture. Watching the abdomen rise and fall, quickly but as you grow with the posture it become more controlled

- Stay here for about 10—15 seconds initially. You will feel the thighs burn as they work hard to maintain the Bridge

- The legs are the foundation in this posture. You will feel the buttocks tightening. This is a great posture pre-holiday! It tones up the buttocks and gets rid of cellulite

The back is fully arched and so space is created in the spinal discs bringing release from tension in the whole back. The thyroid is massaged, the neck opened and extended so this eases headaches. The buttocks are toned and legs working strong, excellent for cellulite and to tone the legs and thigh area. It is also a very good posture for those going through the Menopause as it activates the Thymus gland and opens up the chest area helping to release, as with all Yoga postures, stagnant energy within the body.

<u>To come out of the posture:</u>

- Gently release the buttocks to the ground, very slowly and controlled. Come down as if you were releasing the back to the floor vertebrae by vertebrae, one at a time until you are back lying down fully.

- The tailbone being the last bit to reach the floor.
- Release the legs, now lying back in Corpse pose.

It is important to do a counter pose after a posture such as the Bridge, which has extended and arched the back one way. So now we need to relax the back the other way. Here's a few counter poses to remember:

COUNTER POSES

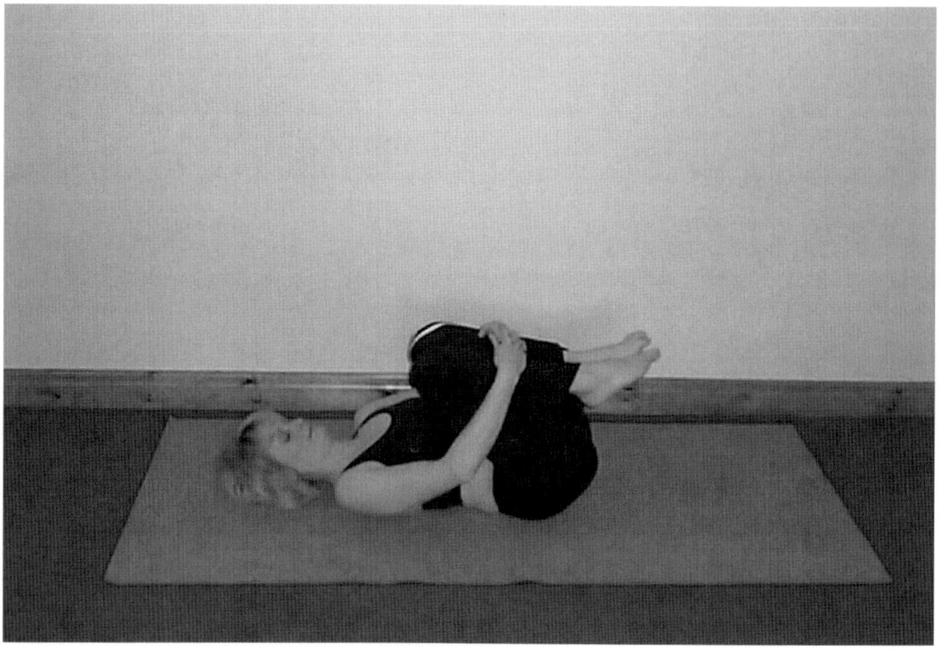

Counter Pose

- After completing Bridge posture, lying flat, bring the knees gently up into the chest and exhale, bringing the head towards the knees.
- Hold for count of 1—4 as you exhale and inhale as you release back to the floor, and then repeat, knees still bent, bring them into the body and exhale as you take the body back down.
- As you exhale allow the body to soften as you take the head to the knees. This pose relaxes the back as in the previous posture it was arched the opposite way.

This posture softens the back as it releases into the floor as you bring the knees up, the neck and head relax as you bring the forehead to the knees. Remember to work at your own pace with all postures. You might find in the beginning your head does not reach your knees but as the back relaxes and as your body opens up to the posture it will become easier. This posture is also good for trapped wind/gas!

Our spine houses many nerves. Postures such as the Bridge and the counter pose exercise the spine and massage the discs, vertebrae and nerve endings. This brings a fresh supply of blood to the whole spine and all the cells, nerves and muscles are rejuvenated. Not a lot of people realise that this is the beauty of Yoga. It is not just performing the postures but what internal action these postures have on our body.

CHILD'S POSE

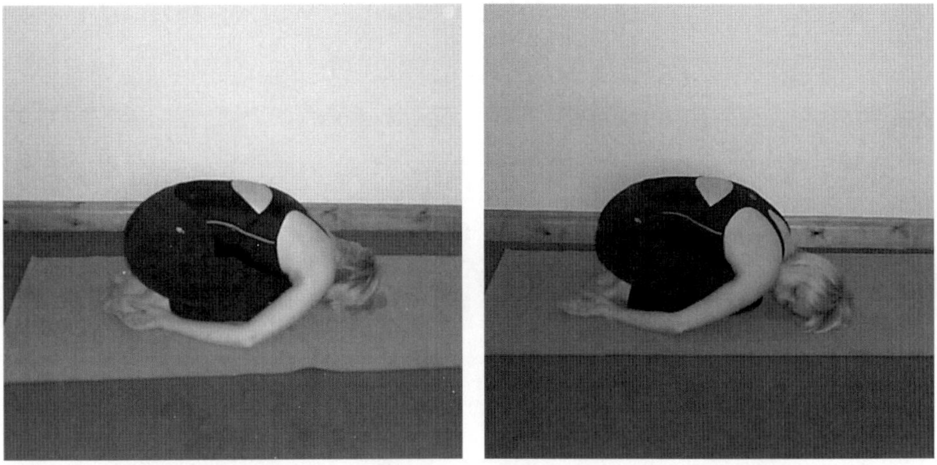

Child's Pose (Counter Pose/relaxation pose)

- To perform this pose sit back on your heels, knees against the floor, so you are kneeling, buttocks on heels
- Take the arms out round the sides of the body, hands resting near feet, neck to side, head resting on floor either directly in front of knees or to the side, whichever is more comfortable
- Staying in the posture allow the back to open up, the groin and hips to soften. Your breathing should be gentle and the body very relaxed

I find this pose is not only good for relaxing and taking a breather after stronger postures but also great for lower backache or during the menses when you get the dull ache/throbbing sensation. Close your eyes and allow your body to unwind and relax.

This pose relaxes the abdomen and you can use this if you suffer from pain during menstruation. It's also a very calming pose. It brings comfort to the abdomen and intestines. It opens up the lower back and strengthens the hip area. It also allows the spine and neck to release. The heart also getting a good massage as you bend forward and the breath becomes relaxed.

A great counter pose but also a good 'on its own' pose. It also helps you to relax before bedtime if you find it hard to go to sleep. Don't perform this posture straight after food. You should wait 1—2 hours after eating before performing bending forward postures.

LOCUST-(SALAMBASANA)

(Avoid during menstruation)

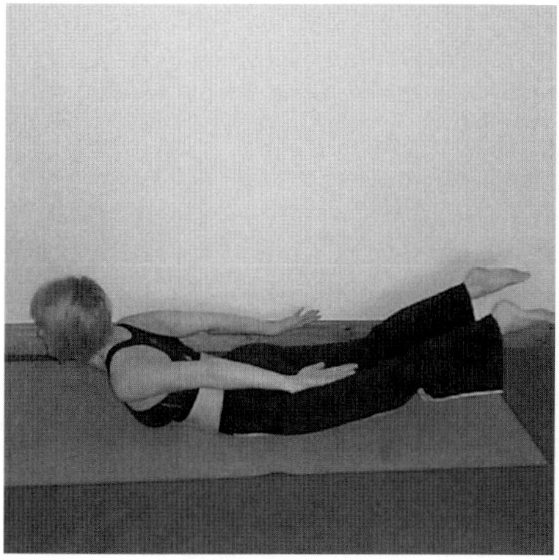

Version 1

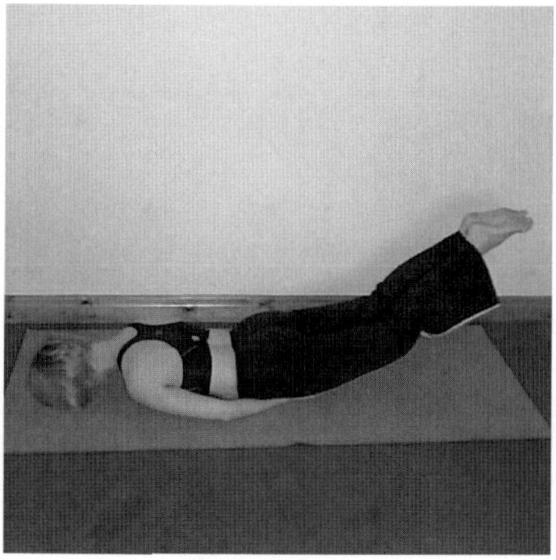

Version 2

This pose really strengthens the back. It has been known to realign the spine and pop discs back into place. It actually helped to strengthen the entire back from the base to the top of the spine near the neck region.

- Lying on the abdomen, flat against the floor, either have the face resting gently on the floor or the head turned to the side, whichever is comfortable.

- Take the hands and place them by the pubic bone, either in a fist shape or just resting by the pubis/lower abdomen. I find making a fist helps and placing the fist firm against the floor. If this feels too uncomfortable just place the palms out flat, against the floor at the side of the body (this way you can use the palms as a lever pushing against the floor). Choose whichever feels comfortable.

- On your inhalation tense the buttocks, forehead against the floor (as in picture), activate the legs, make them strong and pull them tight together and lift, buttocks strong, point the toes and breathe naturally. You are only aiming initially to lift the lower legs up off the floor up to the bottom of the thighs.

- You can keep the forehead on the floor or as in the picture, as you come up on the inhalation, take the arms back, buttocks tight and chest open as you look forward.

- Stay for a count of 5 seconds initially and exhale as you release back to the ground, turning the head to the side and resting, as this is a strong posture.

- You may notice your belly button/lower abdomen pulsating, this is your energy centres energising with the pose.

- This is an excellent pose for the abdomen and reproductive organs. It tones the liver and spleen and rejuvenates the whole spine. The buttocks are activated and toned along with the legs.

- Avoid this pose whilst menstruating. I have found it is best to let the body rest during the menses and avoid any postures that are too strenuous. Although this posture does have a relaxing affect on the reproductive organs. I have found whilst practising this posture only once or twice a week it really does help with PMS and abdominal pain. It also tones up the stomach muscles and lower back.

THE BOW

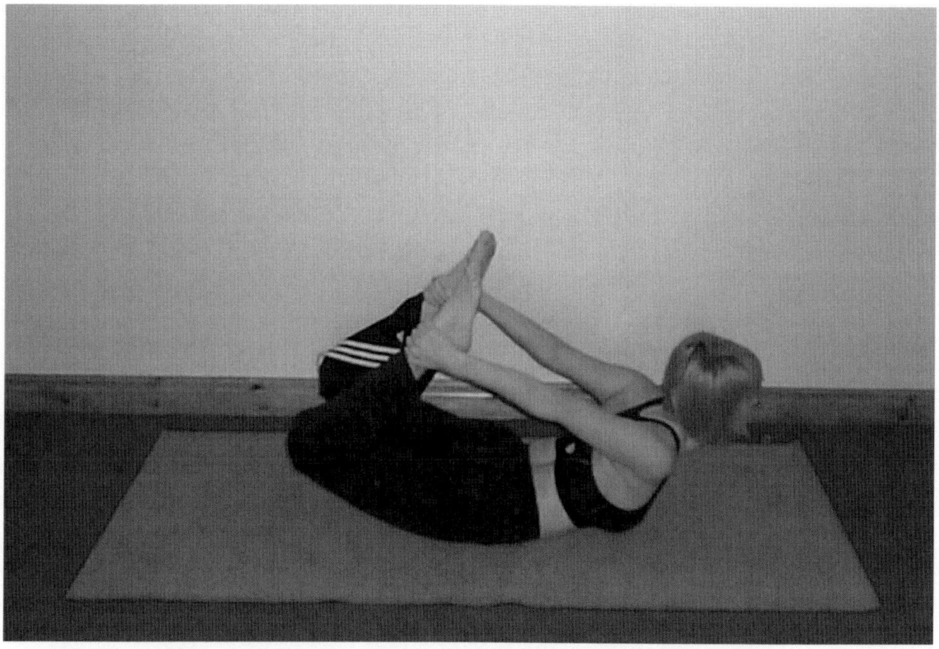

Bow Posture - Avoid during Menstruation

A real exhilarating and strong posture. It works on the lower energy centres and massages the abdomen and brings fresh blood supply to this area. You can actually feel the belly button and lower abdomen pulsate in this posture as in Locust. This pulsating shows you the energy centre is activated. This pose is very beneficial if you are feeling a little run down. It energises your whole body and is very invigorating. It's one of those postures you should do when you don't feel like doing any exercise! How you will feel after will be evidence that the posture is working, it will really wake you up!

- To perform this posture, lie flat against the floor, head to one side. Arms relaxed against the floor by the sides of the body

- On your next inhalation get ready to take the arms down by the ankles as you bring the legs up bent, take hold of the ankles, forehead on floor

- Then when ready inhaling and lifting up, pushing the legs away, the hands grip the ankles, kind of like a lever. The arms are pulled back, shoulder blades work strong

- The chest is opened fully (excellent for asthmatics!) neck relaxed, looking forward. Hold the posture in the beginning for 2—5 breaths. You can breathe naturally when you are up in the posture

- The breath will be rapid to start but work to control the breath and you will control your stamina and work with it to stay stronger and longer in the posture

- To come down, exhale gently as you release the ankles and release the torso to the floor, chest, arms, and then head, turning to the side, at this point build up your lungs. That is take in a few breaths as you relax down, building up your reservoir of energy

- When you are ready, take hold of the ankles and come into the posture again. Feel the stomach area pulsating, notice how the whole body feels, the tension releasing, the shoulders opening, the lower back working, the buttocks strong and tense as you hold in the posture

Repeat 3—4 times initially. Taking that all-important rest in between. Building up your energy with the breath, inhaling deep into the lungs. This is a strong posture. It can follow on from the Locust posture. This way you can make up your routines so you become familiar with the postures. As you become more flexible and open up you can try lifting the legs higher so the thighs come off the floor! This happens as the back opens up and becomes stronger as you utilise all the back muscles and strengthen each vertebra and muscle along the spine.

COBRA

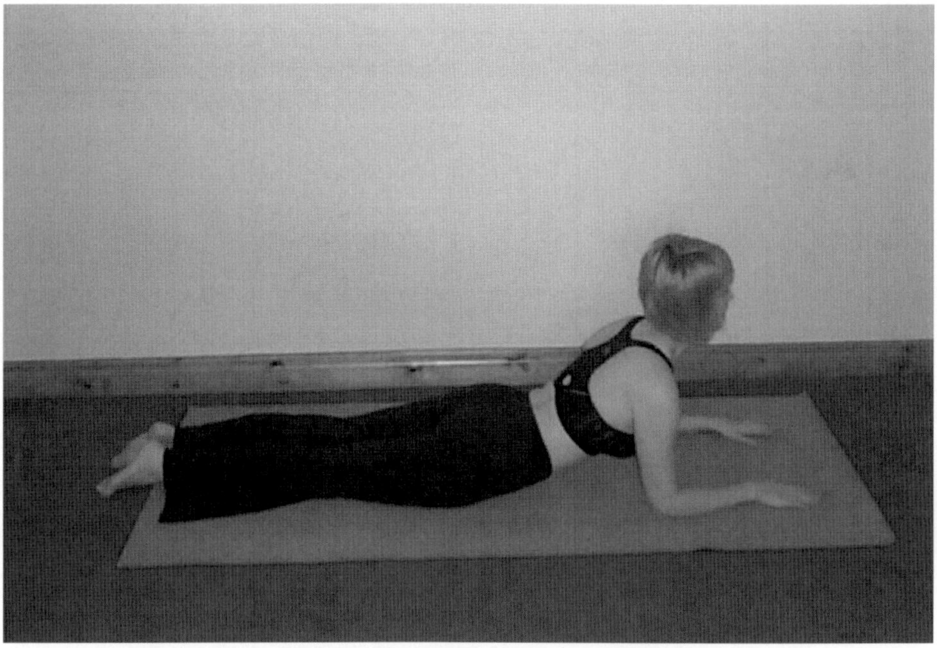

Side View Cobra - Avoid during Menstruation

Front View Cobra - Avoid during Menstruation

<u>How to do Cobra:</u>

- Lying down, forehead on floor, place the hands just up from the shoulders on the floor, shoulder width apart
- Bringing the head up gently, keeping the chin against the floor, lift the top of the body up, using the hands to pressurise against the floor (like a lever)
- Lifting the chest off the floor gently, shoulders light, come up only up to the belly button, this should remain against the floor. Keep the hips firmly against the floor
- The back strong, the buttocks activated (tensed and strong)
- Now look forward, breathing naturally, think about lengthening the spine, allowing it to open up
- Keep the arms pressurising into the floor, the arms outstretched straight in front, looking forward. You should be breathing naturally throughout this posture
- You may feel the stomach pulsating again, right behind the belly button, this is the energies mentioned earlier

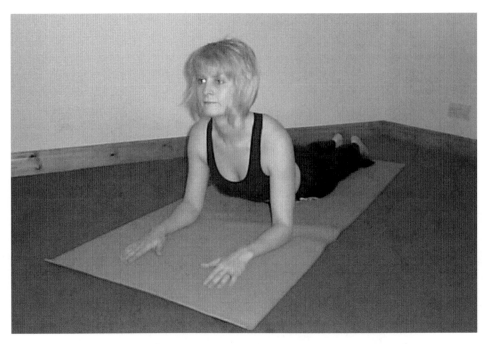

- To come down, exhale, then gently release the body down, taking the arms to the sides of the body, as you relax against the floor, turning the head to the side and resting

- Aim at staying up for 10—30 seconds initially

- To come back into the posture take the hands underneath the shoulders and pressurise the hands against the floor, fingers facing forwards, inhale and lift up back into cobra

- Don't forget to activate the buttocks and pressurise the hands and forearms, this helps to keep you up in the pose

This posture opens up and rejuvenates the entire spine. You may find initial discomfort found at the lower back at the sacral region. This is where many Endo sufferers will get a lot of pain. It is where the Parasympathetic Nervous System is located and this is very active for those with Endo. This is due to imbalances in and around this area due to the body often working against itself and the nerves giving out signals as the body is in pain.

This posture will help immensely as it brings a fresh supply of blood to the whole spine. It can help to ease pain in between discs and with regular practice can realign the spine. The hips open, the chest opens and the shoulders are light, no tension.

Going off on a tangent slightly I wanted to bring your awareness to the importance of:

<u>Parasympathetic Nervous System:</u>

(The Parasympathetic Nervous System is concerned with conservation and restoration of energy, as it causes a reduction in heart rate and blood pressure, and facilitates digestion and absorption of nutrients, and consequently the excretion of waste products).

Many women may experience headaches and neck pain about a week before the onset of their period. This has to do with the Parasympathetic Nervous System, located along the spine from the base to the top of the neck. Briefly, I just wanted to point out a possible cause for these headaches, a week before the onset of the period the body begins to prepare itself to release toxins. This is why it is a good idea to note down when your periods are and how you feel. For instance, in my case every 2nd cycle, my right tube is slightly blocked so I know that 2nd cycle is going to be quite painful. Your cycle changes every month, one month the left ovary will be dominant, the next cycle it will be the right ovary. My Naturopath told me this and I really didn't know anything about this, it is very valuable information to which I want to share.

So when I get the neck pains I know that it is time to use my castor oil packs with a hot water bottle. This soothes the nerves in the neck, face and eyes as I sometimes feel my eyeballs are going to pop out! The pain can be similar to neuralgia, twinges in the head and neck, the face feeling tingly and tight. This is because the body is all wired up. It is trying to perform a function and the body is so very tense. The Castor oil packs are a godsend. I now have to use these 2—3 times a week especially the week before my period as it helps to prepare the body. I don't feel frightened with this pain any more. I know what it is and how to deal with it and again, I want to point out the importance of hot water bottles and castor oil packs. I use a bit of pure wool and Muslim cloth as it helps to soak in the castor oil, but I guess you could use bandage or a sterile dressing/cloth as long as the hot water bottle is placed directly over the top. The areas to place the packs on are:

- Back of the neck
- Lower abdomen
- Lower back
- Upper chest, Thymus area
- Breasts

You can buy Castor Oil form Health stores or by looking on the Internet. It is not too expensive. Use the packs with the Epsom Salt baths (Magnesium baths that I will cover later. Magnesium is needed to combat pain in the body). If you only take one thing away with you from this book please use the Castor Oil packs and Epsom salts. Also try Baking Soda in the bath as this helps to eliminate infection and bacteria in the skin and is lovely to bathe in. Your skin feels really clean. I have found this has also helped my dry skin.

When I have this pain the only thing that works is the packs. They are very soothing and I have found my cycle the following week is easier after using the packs. They kind of prepare the body and make the cycle a whole lot easier. Try this and see.

Now let's get back to Yoga:

DOWNWARD DOG

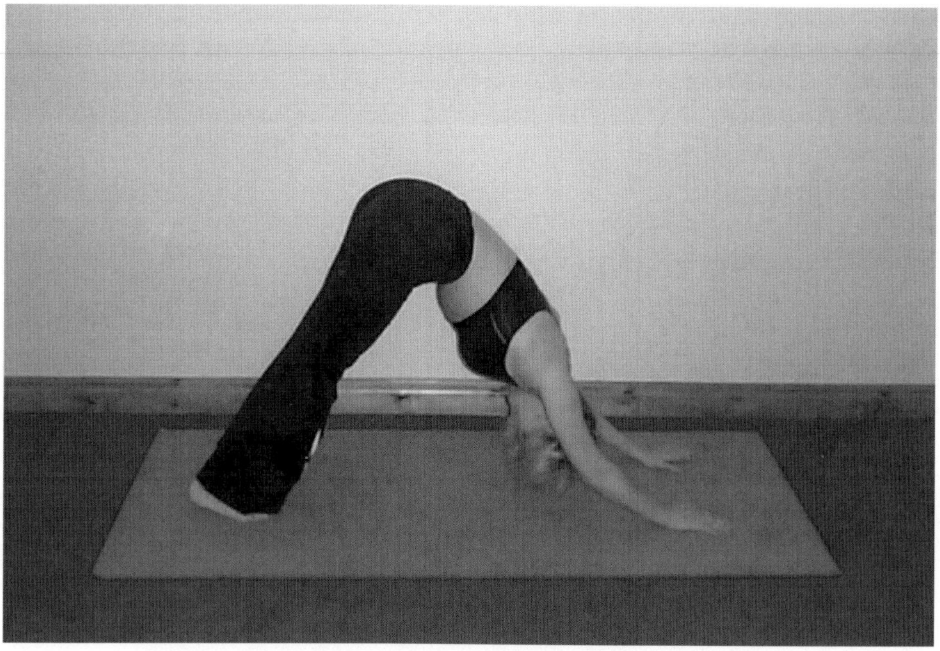

Dog Posture - Avoid during Menstruation

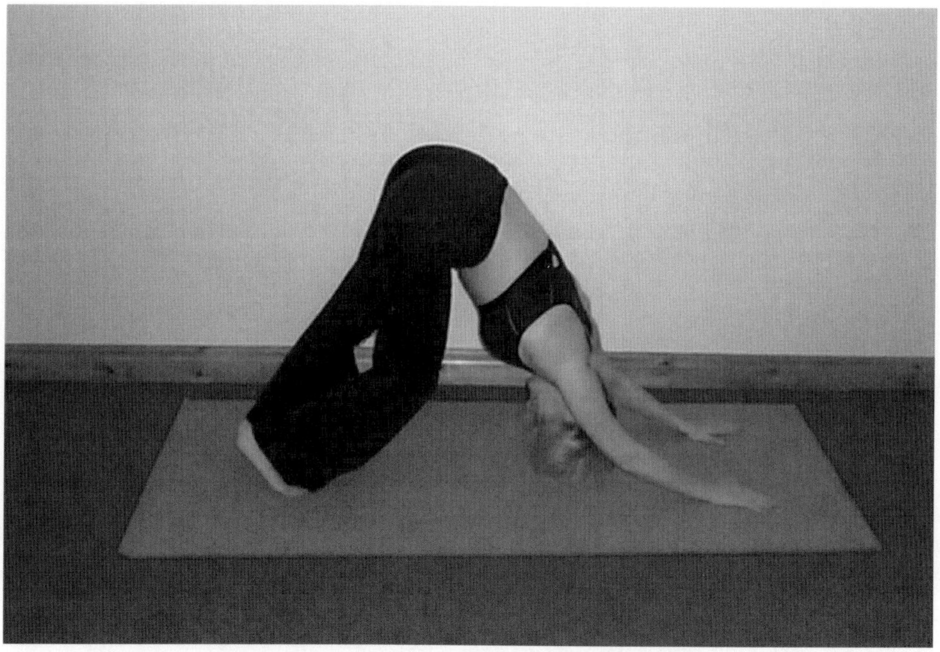

Dog Stretch Variation - Avoid during Menstruation

- It is best to start this posture from on all fours. Inhale and then exhale, sit back on the heels take the arms outstretched in front (arms should be shoulder width apart and stretched out in front of the body say 1—2 ft

- This should not feel uncomfortable so don't stretch too far)

- Still exhaling push the buttocks up to the ceiling as you straighten the legs. The feet should be hip width apart. You can shuffle about in the first stages until you get used to it but this is how you should be:

- Feet hip width apart

- Arms outstretched in front about 1—2 ft away from the body

- Legs strong and stretched

- Feet not against the floor but the heels pushing back feeling the pull and stretch on the hamstrings. In time you may be able to work to get your feet flat on the floor but this will come with practice and flexibility

- Arms are the strong point and locked at the elbow, opening and elongating the arms

- Hands flat on the floor, fingers outstretched and space between each finger, press the hands firmly against the floor as this is your foundation

- Press the toes firmly into the floor as the hands and feet take the weight, they are the building block, foundation

- Think of lifting the hips up to the ceiling creating space

- Let the head and neck be light, allow the head to hang down between the arms

- The shoulders should be squared, taken back not rounded, take the shoulders back a little so they open up, again creating space

- Try and bring the chin gently into the notch in the chest, no tension, just passive, if you cannot manage don't push too hard, just let the head hang but if you can bring the chin slightly into the chest, looking at the stomach and flatness of the thighs

- Work the legs, pull up from the knees, feel the muscles working. If you have knee problems work slowly with this

- (Dog Variation as above) You can bend each knee one at a time to ease tension in the hip and groin area, left, then right, left then right, turning the toes in so you kind of twist and bend the knee forward

- Keep your balance. Remember to push the buttocks up as if you are aiming them at the ceiling, creating space

- Allow the back to soften, lengthen and strengthen

- Breathing natural during the pose

- Duration—10—30 seconds to start with, working up to 3 minutes

This posture will work the whole of the body. It is said that if the head is lower than the heart, as it is in this posture, the heart will receive a good massage. This postures builds up the muscles in the spine and helps to lengthen and ease pressure on spinal discs/vertebrae. It builds up the leg muscles and helps with tension in the neck and shoulder area.

Come into **Child's Pose** to relax.

CHILD'S POSE (with variation)

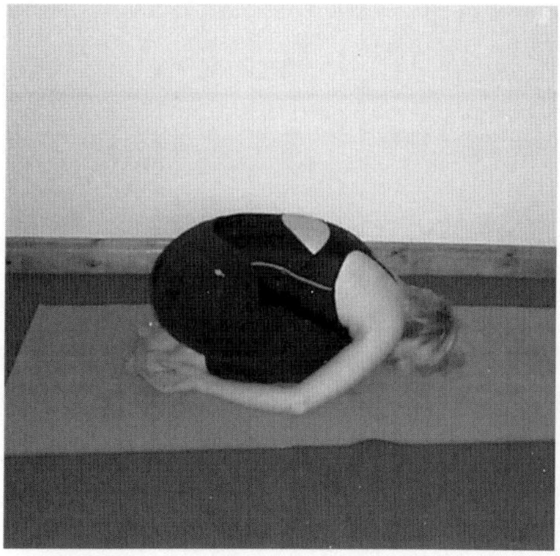

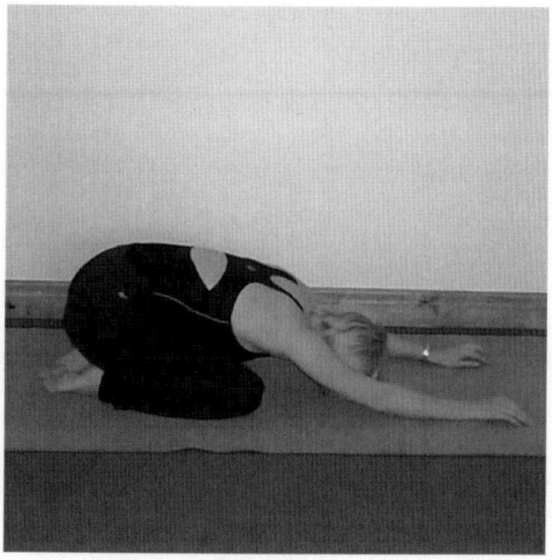

- From Dog above—bring the buttocks back down to the heels, take the arms by the sides of the body

- Place the forehead on the floor to rest or turn it gently to the side

- Allow the back to soften and rest as you rest the buttocks on the heels. Natural breathing, listen and notice how you feel

This is a counter pose so we are allowing the body to rest in between postures.

COMING BACK INTO DOG POSE

- When you are ready to go into dog again take the head looking forward
- Place the hands outstretched, shoulder width apart in front of the body and then come onto toes
- When ready inhale then on the exhalation push the buttocks up into the air, aiming for the ceiling, legs strong and stretched now and pressing the hands firmly into the floor
- Locking the arms, head relaxed between the arms and stay in dog for as long as you feel comfortable. Remember to work with the breath. The deeper the breath the more control you will have.

The Dog Posture is a very invigorating posture and in time you will build up stamina. It exercises the whole body. The head is lower than the heart so the heart will receive a lovely massage. Fresh energy and blood is brought to many organs and they are also massaged. This posture helps to rid the body of toxins as you are bending and holding the pose. Remember to drink plenty of water after practice to flush out toxins.

<u>CAT POSTURE</u>

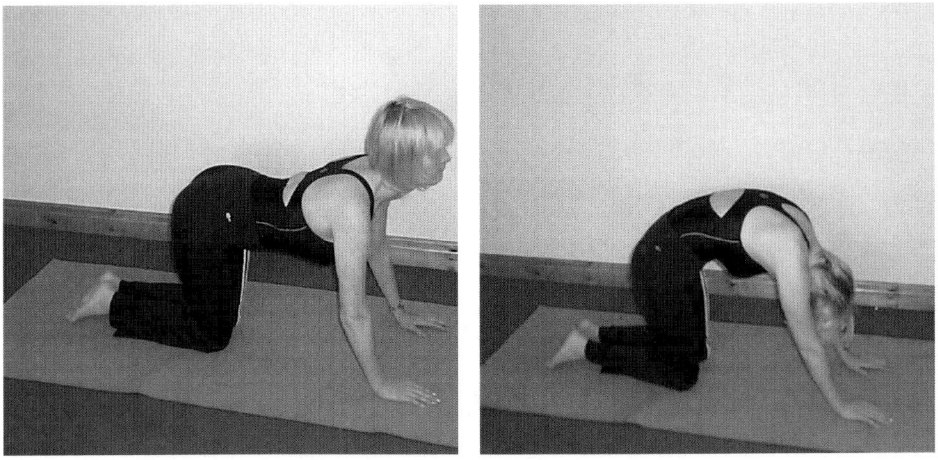

Cat Posture

- Standing on all fours, like a cat. looking forward
- Hands are shoulder width apart placed right out in front, don't overstretched
- Knees bent, feet are hip width apart
- Looking forward, inhaling, chest open, shoulders relaxed
- Point the chin out, opening the neck

- Arms fully outstretched, fingers spread flat against the floor, palms outstretched

- Concave/drop the back so it dips as you push the buttocks away and feel the stretch

- Now get ready to exhale and as you do so you are going to take the chin into the chest, arching the back up to the ceiling

- Push out from the shoulder blades, really push the back up the ceiling, chin into notch in chest or as best you can, you are now folding in position as you exhale

- Ready to inhale we drop the spine, open up and look forward, chin out, chest wide, shoulders relaxed, arms still stretched out in front. Feel the stomach stretch, the whole of the body stretches.

What you are trying to get used to here is the opening and closing action, the rolling rhythm of the spine. Imagine a ball at the top of the spine as you exhale, you close up; the back is arched, as you exhale the spine drops, you open up the ball rolls down the spine to the buttocks. Get used to this rhythm, exhaling, closing up, inhaling opening up, and stretching the buttocks away. This is an excellent posture for keeping the spine active.

If you want to rest then just drop down into Child's Pose. Sit back on the heels, the hands outstretched in front and take the forehead to the floor. Allow the back to soften. When you are ready to go back into the posture inhale and come back on all fours and begin again, inhaling, etc.

Work with this posture and wave like motion opening, closing for about 3 minutes.

You can enhance this posture by doing a side stretch.

- When on all fours gently walk the both hands round to the left so you face the buttocks on the left side

- Then walk them round to the right, looking towards the right buttock. Feel the lovely stretch.

This tones the abdomen and hips/waistline and really helps to bring vitality back into the spine. It brings back flexibility in the spine and is also a great posture if you have a headache or shoulder/neck tension as the motion of the spine works to release the upper and lower back, neck and shoulders.

Remember the Counter Pose, sitting back on the heels and outstretch the arms, forehead to floor and rest. In time your hips, waist and spine will open up and the rhythm of the spine opening and closing will become easier. There may be initial discomfort but this is due to calcification in the neck and shoulder area and will cease with regular practice. What you are achieving with this posture is bringing about the natural rhythm of the spine, massaging the nerves and cells along the spinal column, which brings about many benefits.

Boat Posture

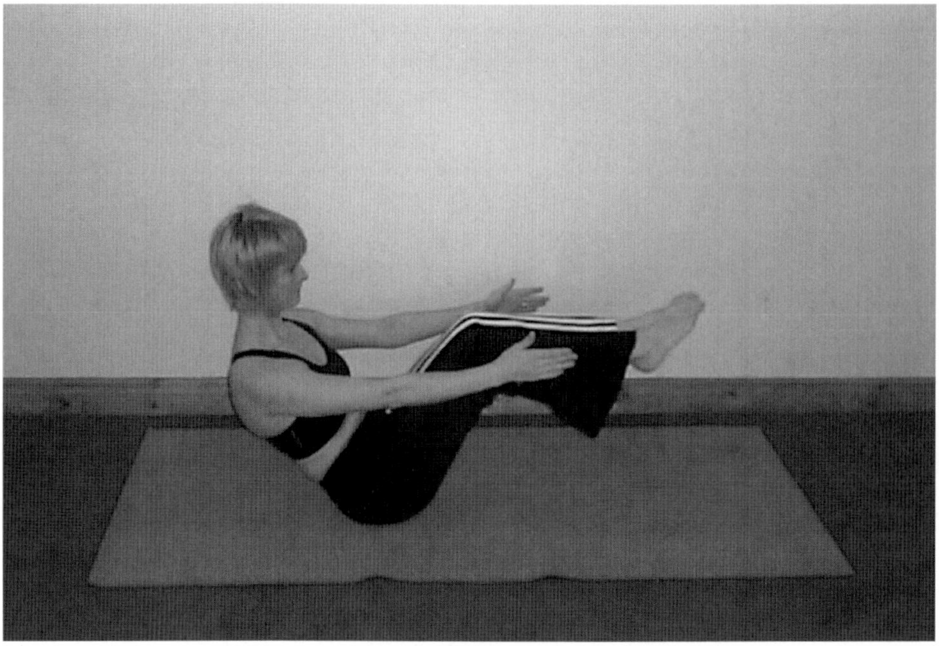

Boat Posture

An excellent posture for building up stomach muscles and toning the arms, thighs and legs. Helps with stamina and getting rid of excess energy, when you really feel like a good work out! Here goes:

To perform this posture:

- Sit on the floor with legs outstretched in front of you
- Take the balance by placing the arms either side of the body, hands pressed against floor
- When ready lean back slightly, not too much and take the fingertips to the floor
- On the inhalation take the legs together as you lift them up knees slightly bent, feet together
- Take the arms up parallel to the knees, palms facing knees, fingers pointing forward, and together
- The knees should be gently brought up towards the chest and pull the stomach in tight
- The legs working strongly, notice the thigh muscles and abs working strong
- Don't lean too far back just enough to gain balance as in the picture above

- Stay in pose for 5—10 seconds, working within your own limitations. As you progress you can work up to 20—30 seconds

- To relax out of the pose bring the knees into the chest and wrap the arms round the knees, hugging the knees tightly into the chest, back tall, straight and erect

- When ready to go into the pose again just release the knees, take the fingertips to the floor to balance, leaning back slightly and then take the legs into position as shown above

- Do 4 reps. Pose—rest—pose –rest etc

Each time you go into the pose itself, work on staying a little longer than previously, this is how you build up stamina. In the initial stages of practising this posture you may feel a slight burning sensation as you work the thighs. This is just working on toning up the muscles. The key is to work with the breath. Inhaling, exhaling and softening the breath. The key to staying in the posture, is learning to work with your breathing. Work to control the breath as you are up in the posture, when you want to come down, just release down and hug the knees into the chest. Notice how your body feels, that's very important to!

Fish Posture:

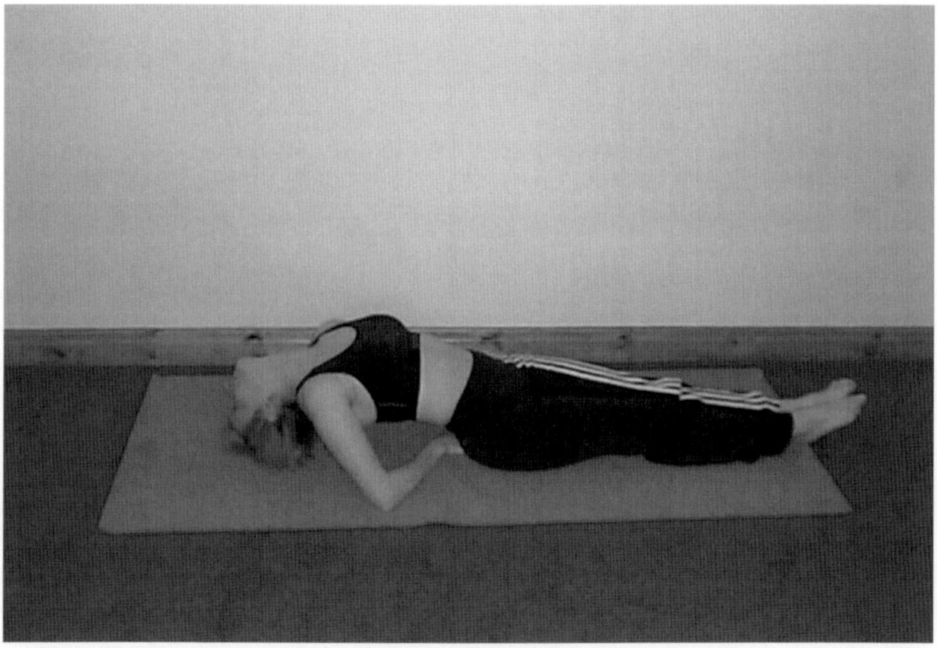

Fish Posture

This is a wonderful posture for opening up the whole back, shoulders and chest. It also works on the

Thyroid gland in the neck as the neck is gently stretched backwards. Work with this slowly to start with. This posture can help to regulate hormones, working on balancing from within and helping mood swings and PMS symptoms. Work slowly with this one. Many people don't like to take the head back, as is done in this posture but, again, work slowly and it will become a familiar posture.

If you want to take a pillow behind the head, to place the top of the head on when you go back (as shown in the photo) then please do. In time you will be able to open up, opening the chest, arching the back and releasing the head, naturally to the floor. In the initially stages the breathing can be quite rapid but just work slowly, staying in the posture for a few breaths initially, coming out controlled and gently, this is very important.

<u>How to do:</u>

- Lying in Corpse pose, gently place the hands underneath the lower back, by the top of the buttocks
- You can place the hands here or make fists and place these under the lower back
- Now as you inhale gently shuffle the torso forward, moving the legs forward as you come up on your elbows
- Looking down at the feet, natural breathing, inhale and on the next exhalation take the head back and place the top of the head against the floor, work with this slowly
- The aim is to have the top of the head resting on the floor
- The chest begins to open and expands with the breathe
- The upper back is now arched over, opening the chest, and bringing the shoulder blades together
- Feel the stretch in the neck area
- Allow the breathing to be natural, it may feel strange at first but work with inhaling and exhaling gently, don't harness the breath
- To come up gently bring the head up, slowly, take the hands out from the lower back and place them at the sides of the body
- Releasing back down to Corpse pose.

It is important to do a Counter pose here so from Corpse pose, take a few breaths and then bring the knees into the chest:

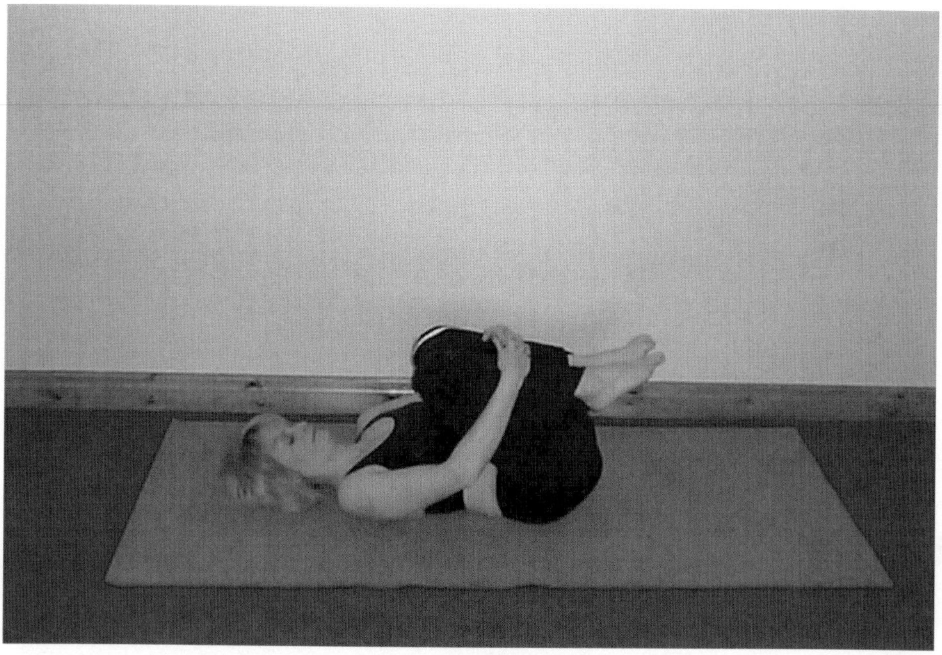

Counter Pose

Remain here for a minute or two then release the legs and go back into Fish. The counter pose works the back in the opposite direction. Repeat the Pose and then counter pose 3 times. Pay particular attention to the breathing movement in the chest and abdomen when you are in Fish. It really is an exhilarating and very opening posture. Great for Asthmatics and those who may have problems with the Thyroid Gland.

Extended Forward Bend

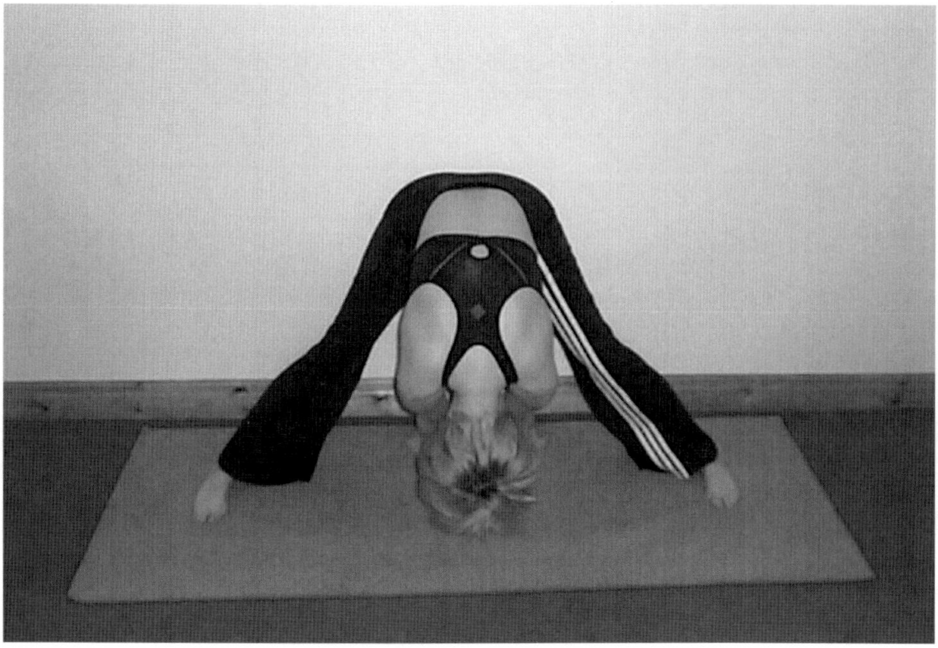

Extended Forward Bend

This is another strong stretch, opening and lengthening the spine. Bringing flexibility to the hamstrings and abductor muscles. Work slowly initially. With practice the flexibility and lengthening in the spine will come.

- Standing with feet together jump them/or shuffle them to 3 ½ to 4 feet apart, wide stance
- Hands on waist, think about lengthening from the waist upwards, natural breathing
- The feet should be pressed firmly into the ground as this is your foundation in the pose, what is going to help you balance
- Toes pointing forward, press the feet firmly, all flat against the floor
- Looking forward, and release the hands to the floor, if you are on fingertips that's fine, work within your limitations, fingertips/palms to floor
- Now lift the head and look forward, we are working and elongating the spine here, opening and lengthening
- Remain for 5—10 seconds

- Now as you exhale work on dropping the torso between the legs, looking down at the floor, moving the upper body down to the floor as in the picture above. Focus on the lower back, this is where we are working on lengthening from

- Remember legs and feet—foundation—keep the legs firm and strong, lock the knees, work the legs strongly in this pose. Pressurise the feet into the floor. So the bottom of the body working strongly, the top half of the body, the torso, arms and head are light and soft and lengthening

- Work with the breath in this pose, as you inhale allow the energy to enter the body, as you exhale let the spine release further bringing your head closer to the floor

- Pull in the stomach muscles, creating space to bend and open

- Remain for 20—30 seconds and to come up, place the fingers/palms on the floor, looking forward, hold for a second or two

- Take hands on waist/hips and gently come up to centre

- Repeat when you are ready to go into it again, focus on lower back releasing, legs strong, working on lengthening and softening the spine

A great posture for developing the hamstring and abductor muscles. It increases digestive powers. These standing postures help those who want to lose weight. Its also very calming when the head is lower than the heart as it is in this posture and great for the back to, taking pressure off the discs and opening the whole back. The legs are also toned in this posture. Just work slowly with it and remember it involves using the hamstrings so don't hyperextend (stretch too far with legs and knees). With regular practice you will be able to get your head on the floor and take the arms back further between the legs. It's a beautiful posture.

Forward Bend

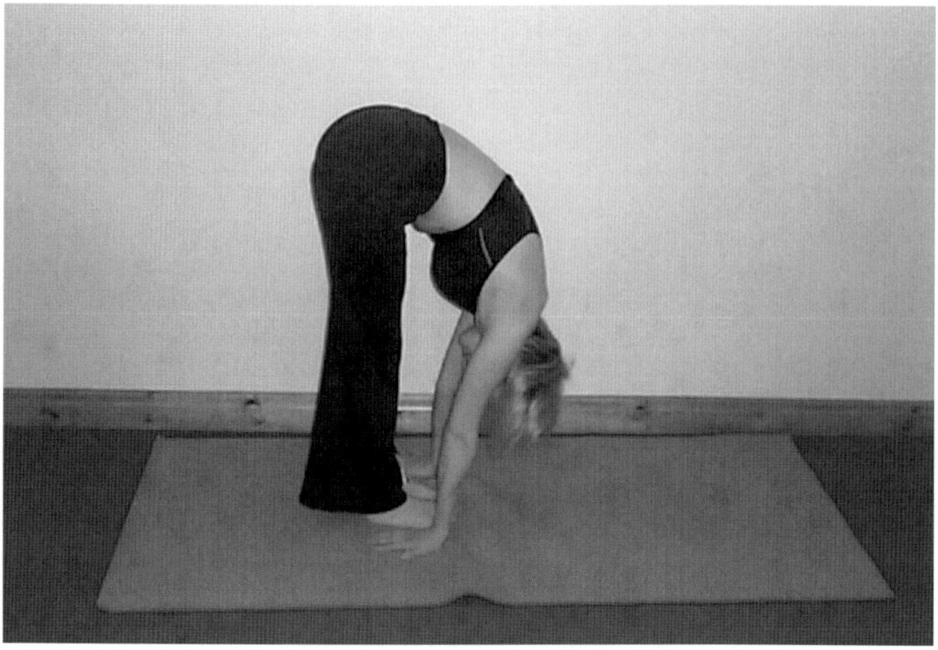

Forward Side Stretch

I have heard many a Yoga Teacher say "If you only ever learn one Yoga posture this has to be it"! A great opening posture, tones the whole back, legs and the head and neck relaxed and lengthening. The abdominal muscles are toned and the digestive juices increased, bringing energy to the stomach area, toning, energising and revitalising the internal organs. The head is lower than the heart so the heart receives a good massage. The liver and spleen are activated in this posture and this helps with cleansing and removing stagnant energy around these organs. This pose can also help with slipped discs in the back, the opening and lengthening action creates space for the discs to move/open/relax.

How to do:

- Standing tall, feet about hip width apart, gently tilt the pelvis forward so the body is in line, the buttocks gently rolled underneath by gently bringing the hips slightly forward and up
- Inhaling and lengthening from the hips. Allow the front of the body to open as you stand tall
- Gently roll the chin into/towards the notch in the chest, opening up the back of the neck
- Now begin on the exhalation to roll the body down gently, hands on thighs and as you roll down allow the arms to move down the thighs, knees, shins
- If you can only reach knees that's fine just stay there

- If your hands are moving forward further to the feet then place the hands on the floor as in picture
- Let the head be light, neck light, back lengthening
- Pull in the stomach/abs and begin to create space between the stomach and thighs, imagine you are leaning over a freshly painted fence with your best dress on! You don't want to get paint on it so really pull in the stomach muscles/abs and create space
- You can interlock the elbows, take hold of opposite elbows if you prefer, let the head hang between the arms, the arms then act as a weight. Remember not to overstretch and work within your own capabilities
- Breathing should be natural with this posture, using the exhalation to lengthen further and stretch. You may begin to feel the body getting longer, opening up
- To come out of this posture release the arms, let them be floppy, chin still in notch in chest gently begin to roll back up vertebrae by vertebrae, like the cog on a bike chain, rolling the body back up to standing
- You might want to rotate the shoulders a little and take the ear towards the left shoulder, back to centre, and then take right ear towards right shoulder to release the neck area
- When ready go into the posture again as outlined above, working on stretching and opening
- You can use blocks under the hands to help you if you cannot reach the floor, or if it is too intense a stretch on the lower back

A wonderful rejuvenating posture that I have personally found clears the head. When we get stressed and tired, tension builds up and we want to just hang loose and let it go—this posture is excellent when you feel like this. This posture can be used when menstruating but remember that many of us have pain in the lower back with Endometriosis so just work slowly. The opening up and lengthening in this posture brings many benefits.

Hip/Groin Release Exercise)

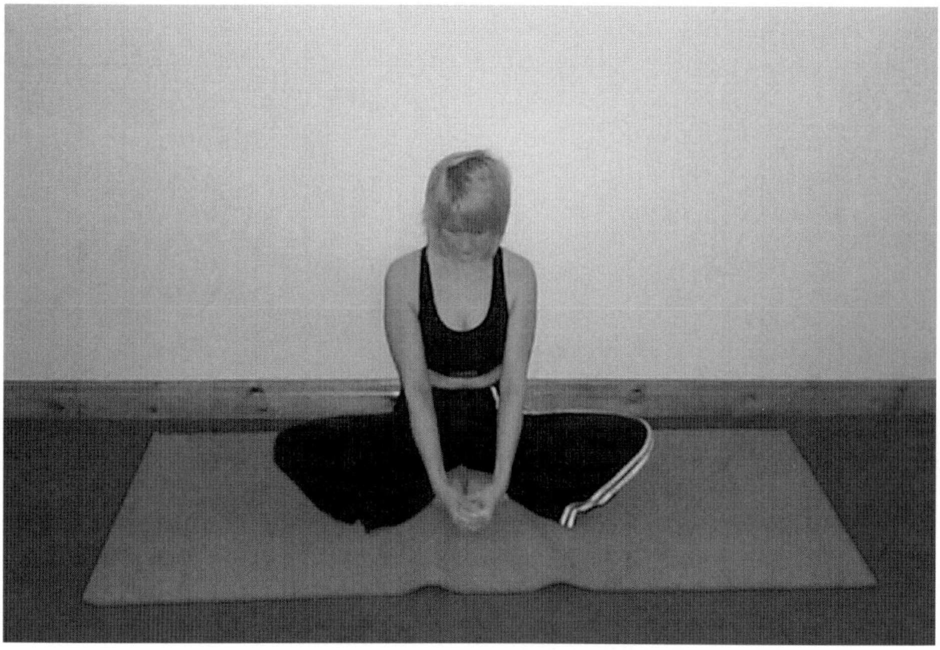

Hip & Groin Release Pose

This posture is great for opening up the hip and groin area. An area so many of us hold a great deal of tension. When we work with this posture the emotions that surface as we release tension and build up can be quite amazing. It is a freeing up feeling of release and brings many benefits.

How to do:

- Sitting tall bring the soles of the feet together so that they press firmly against each other
- At this point if you want to sit on a cushion that's fine, this will help to open the hip area
- From here we are working to push the feet together, and bring them close to the Peritoneum/ groin area
- When you feel comfortable begin to place the elbows against the upper thigh as in picture above. Use the arms/elbows to push the thighs down
- If you can activate the leg muscles and push down also this will help. Inhaling deeply and as you exhale this is when to push down
- Using the exhalation to soften the groin and hip area

Don't force it just allow the breath and arms to work together. Now taking hold of the feet try and push the legs down using the muscles of the legs on their own. No use of hands, push the feet together firmly and this will help you to move the legs down.

- Bring the legs up together to rest, knees bent and hug the knees tightly into the chest. Go into the posture again when you are ready

In the picture I am using both my hands and arms to push down. Try this if you can, it really helps to release the groin and hips.

Work slowly and within your own limitations. When you get some quiet time work with this releasing posture. Sitting tall and working to release the legs, hips and groin.

Please do not perform this posture if you have just had surgery as it really does open up the lower areas of the body so work slowly.

Cobbler Pose

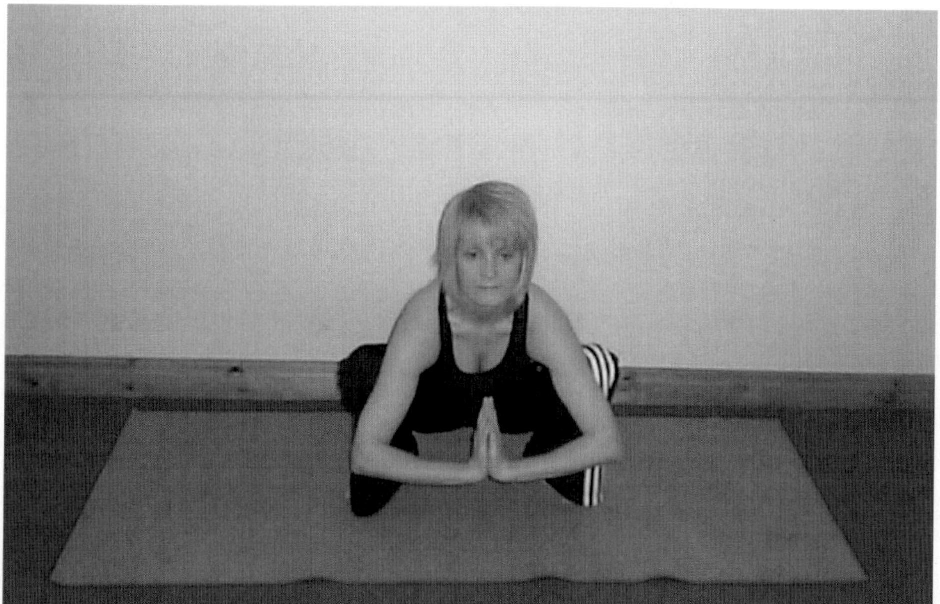

Cobbler Pose

A lot of Indian ladies use this posture to help with menstruation discomfort. It helps to keep the bladder and kidneys working, strengthens the uterus and other lower muscles and helps to also ease pelvic discomfort. It opens up the hips and lower back.

How to do:

- Standing tall take the feet about 2 ½ to 3 feet apart, then as you exhale move towards the floor from standing

- Dropping the buttocks between the feet, buttocks are not on the floor, as you can see from the picture above I am sat kind of between my own hips and between the feet. The groin and buttocks aiming towards the floor

- Take the arms and elbows in between the legs, pushing the arms against the knees to widen the pose, creating space in the hip/groin area

- Try and keep the feet flat on the floor. If not this is what you are working towards, the lower back has to soften and release, this will happen in time and the feet will sit naturally flat on the floor

- Push the palms together; this helps when pushing against the knees.

You can bounce if you like! That is you take the buttocks off the legs and back, off and back, just lifting a little away. A really nice posture. You can stay here for as long as you feel necessary. To come up inhale, release the arms and stand tall.

This posture brings a fresh blood flow to the lower extremities, it kind of locks the lower body so all the organs here are massaged and rejuvenated. It helps to ease discomfort in hips, groin, pelvis area and as mentioned can assist with menstrual pain and discomfort. Whilst in the pose you are working to tighten up the lower extremities so pull them up. As if you are stopping yourself going to the loo!

(At this point I will mention that it may be advisable if you are menstruating to perform the postures with a sanitary towel in place rather than a tampon. It doesn't really matter but I find the towel is more comfortable and, as in the pose outlined above there is no risk of the tampon coming out!

Whilst teaching classes whilst menstruating I have worn a tampon but it is entirely up to you. Many women find that they prefer to where baggy clothing such as sweatpants and or joggers when practicing during that time of the month. Many will avoid practising. There is no harm in practising certain Yoga postures when you are bleeding. It depends entirely on how you feel that day. If you want to rest then rest, it's just what your body needs. If you want to practice then practice but avoid the inverted (upside down postures). It is just advisable to do this during the menses.

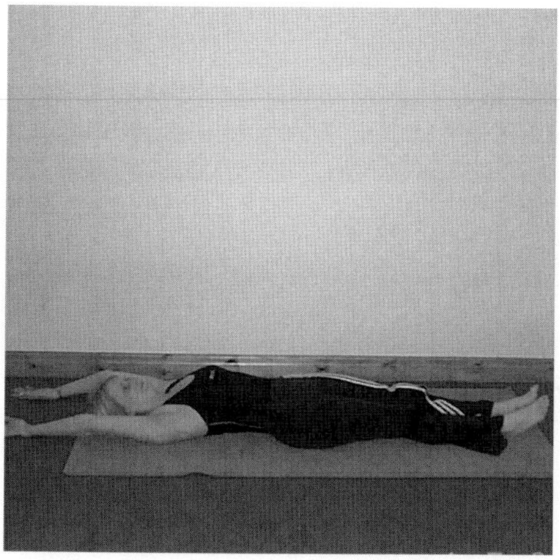

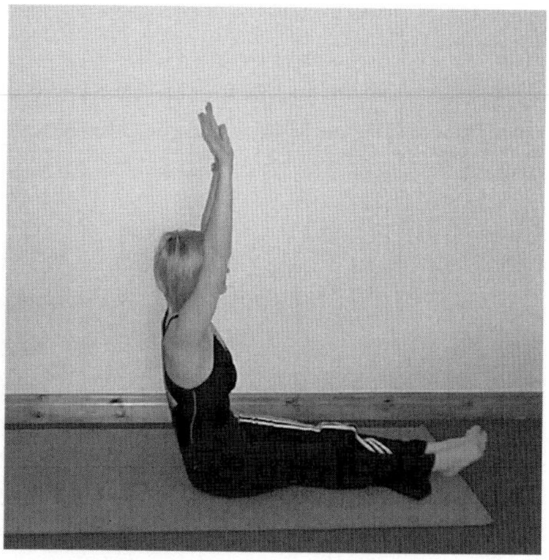

Total Floor Workout

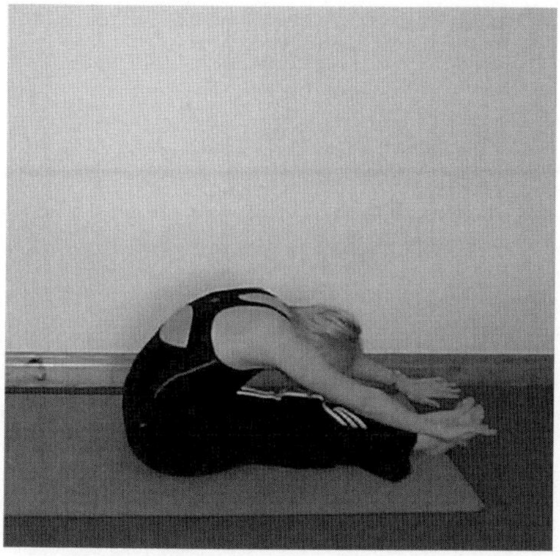

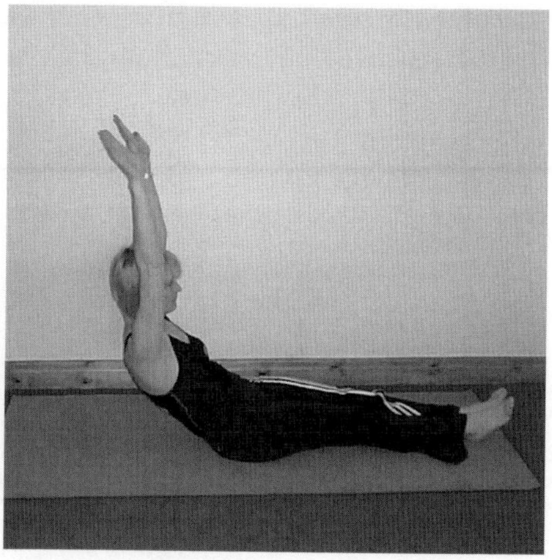

This is a very fluid and rhythmic workout. It involves working with the breath and timing the movement. Give it a go and see how you feel.

- Lying in Corpse pose, allow the body to release against the floor

- On the inhalation sit up to centre, use the hands to pressurise against the floor to push you up if necessary but ideally try and use the abs/stomach muscles

- From centre take a few breaths, then release towards the feet, taking the upper torso, head and arms towards the feet, if you can touch feet great, if not just where you are is ok

- Inhaling up back to centre, using the stomach muscles, keep the legs strong and firm against the floor

- Exhaling now, taking the back slowly towards the floor, as the back reaches the floor, inhale bringing the legs to 90°, feet pointing towards ceiling

- Now exhaling, press the arms into the floor as you lift the buttocks off the ground and take the legs over the head now towards the floor, you can hold the hands on the lower back/buttocks if you wish however you feel comfortable

- Inhaling and now lift the legs back over to 90° angle, toes pointing towards ceiling

- Exhaling taking the legs to the floor gently and controlled, feel the abs working

- This completes one round. The idea is to work faster each time getting a rhythmic movement and using the breath

Lifting up—INHALE
Closing down—releasing—EXHALE

This posture is brilliant for weight management, bringing elasticity to the front and back of the body, working the hip and groin area and strengthening the lower spine. If you don't feel very agile in the beginning it doesn't matter, work slowly and with regular practice you will be able to manage without using the hands.

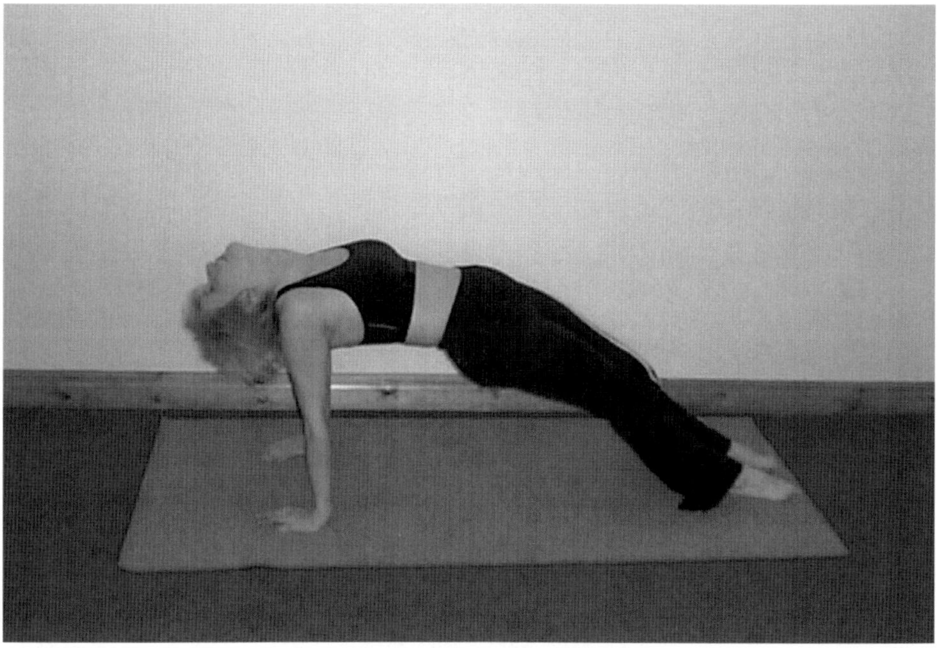

Intense Stretch

This is a pretty strong and energising posture. Remember the Fish pose earlier on, we are putting the head and neck in a similar position, the chest is opened, the arms and legs are strong.

How to do:

- Sit on the floor and take the legs out in front—feet not too far apart
- Take the arms to the sides of the body and point the hands away towards the head as in picture
- Inhale, just looking forward and just practice lifting the buttocks off the floor
- Exhaling down and relax
- Inhaling up, lifting the buttocks, activate them, pull them in tightly, strong holding
- The soles of the feet should move towards the floor as you lift the buttocks up, this is a strong stretch on the ankles as they reach towards the floor so just work slowly. The idea is to get the feet flat on the floor as in the picture. If you prefer just work on the heels and as you slide the torso forward as you come up the feet will move towards the floor, again just work slowly, if still on heels that's fine. The flexibility will come
- Release down
- Once more come up, inhaling, buttocks tight and notice when you come up the torso moves forward, notice the thighs and legs stretching and working strongly
- When you release down relax the arms and the buttocks, and legs, all working strongly so take a breather
- Ok this time, inhaling and pressurise the arms/hands against the floor
- Lifting the buttocks up and high, the legs move forward
- Now gently exhaling, take the head back, remember work slowly
- If on heels just try and work the feet towards the floor
- If soles of feet on floor pressurise them in and work the front of the legs strongly, pushing the ankles forward to move the feet to the floor
- Breathe as naturally as you can in this posture, it may seem a little strange at first and the breathing may be rapid, work with controlling the breath so it is a gentle inhalation, gentle exhalation

- Keep the buttocks strong and arms and hands pressing into the floor
- When you want to come out bring the head and neck forward to centre, gently. Release the buttocks to the floor and take a rest
- Work to stay in the posture 5—10 seconds then releasing
- Come into Child's pose to relax and then go into the posture again

Variation:

You can if you wish bend the knees, so the feet are flat on the floor, pull in the buttocks and then when up in the pose, gently take the head and neck back. Hold for 5—10 seconds and then release back down. This is a slight variation on the above pose and those who don't like the stretching of the ankles in the above outlined posture find working with bent knees easier to perform. Look at the abdomen when you first get in this pose, why? Because as you work with it you will begin to notice how you tone up!

An excellent posture for those with excess energy and/or restless mind. It really builds up stamina, strengthens the legs, thighs, and ankles and works the pressure points on the feet. Taking the neck and head back also works on the Thyroid Gland. It's great for opening the chest and relieving stiffness in the shoulder area. Remember it's a strong one so if you cannot complete it initially just work with coming up and pinching in the buttocks, opening up the chest and lifting. In time you will gradually move on to performing full posture.

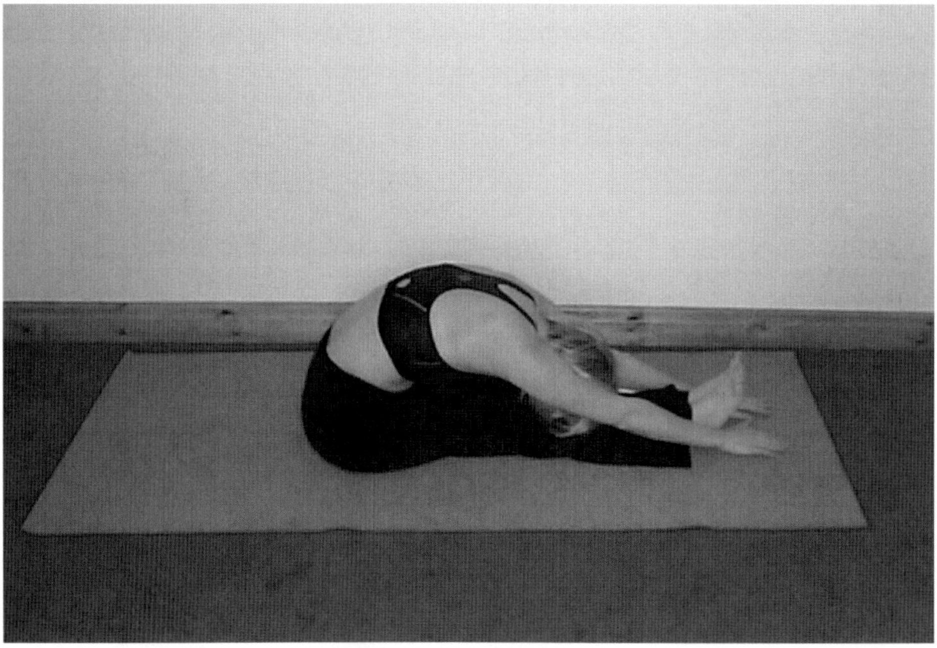

Paschimotasana

This is my favourite Yoga posture. It is not as difficult as it looks. I'll show you how.

How to do:

- Sitting tall, right on top of the buttock bones, looking forward, arms on the thighs
- Inhaling, sitting tall in preparation
- Now bend the knees and sit tall, taking hold behind the knees hugging them into the chest
- Now we are going to move forward, shuffling the feet but keeping the chest as near to the knees/thighs as we can
- So shuffling the feet inch by inch forward, slowly this will bring the upper body with it, your chin will come towards the knees and the body starts to move lower
- Stay with the hugging of the knees and move forward
- You will get to a point where you can release the knees but for now just keep working forward
- Now stop about half way and release the knees, let the legs lie flat out, straighten them and take the hands now behind the calf, looking forward with the head straight, feel the back lengthening
- Still looking forward and working with natural breathe, if you can take hold of the ankles, still looking forward
- Pull in the abdomen and now begin to slowly release the body onto the thighs and release the arms, let the hands rest by the feet
- In the picture above my back could be flattened and lengthened a little more so I would need to look up, concentrating on bringing the kidneys into the back, lifting the back as I look forward and getting that lengthening feeling
- Then I can move forward and will have lengthened a little more
- Work with the breath in this posture, pulling in the abs, exhaling and softening as you exhale
- To come out inhale and looking forward just roll the body back to sitting gently.

Do **Child's Pose** as a counter pose.

Repeat again. This time try this:

- Sitting tall, right on the buttocks again, facing forward, bring the toes towards you to flatten the legs against the floor

- Now take the arms and hands and try and take hold of the big toes, or ankles, wherever you are with flexibility work with that. If hands on knees fine

- Still sitting tall, get a feeling of pulling the back of the spine towards the front of the chest so you are opening up, this creates the space needed to move forward

- Inhaling, get ready

- Exhaling taking gripping onto the big toes, take the head towards the knees and drop the chest onto the thighs

The aim is to get the chest resting on thighs. In time the flexibility will come. Just work with where you are.

- Ok so if chest is on thighs, excellent! Just rest there, watching the breath which will be rapid to start, just work with the breath, softening and working with the exhalation to move the body further against the thighs, softening and lengthening on the exhale is the key.

The longer you remain in the posture the more benefits you will receive.

This posture has a very calming effect on both the breath and the mind, which are very closely linked. This posture will help to bring clarity to mind and aids restful sleep. Another posture where the heart is lower than the head and is thus receiving a good massage. The lower internal organs are massaged, toned and toxins released. This is truly a fantastic posture. Do not become frustrated if you can't bend right forwards, this will come with time. Work within your own limitations and you will soon blossom.

(Make sure you drink 3—4 glasses of water after practice as many of the postures will target organs and you will need to release the toxins out of the system. Water is the best way to do this).

Work with these postures at your own pace, don't rush it, it's not a race. In time your body will develop flexibility and you will also build stamina. Your body will tone and you will also lose weight. Having a bath or hot shower before practice to warm up the muscles really can help you prepare for practice along with the warming up exercises.

This is only a taster of the true and wonderful beauty that is YOGA. I hope that in your own time you will go on to learn more, buy books and find out how this therapy can truly benefit you. Yoga works from the inside out and your body, mind and spirit will reunite bringing harmony, balance and stability.

NAMASTE

SECTION 11
SUN SALUTES

The salute to the Sun exercises all major muscles and joints, and helps you establish a state of calm as you begin and end your day. Centre yourself before you begin (i.e. think calm, think relaxed, focusing on what you are about to do). Stretch slowly and be careful not to strain. Repeat the whole exercise several times alternating legs for better results. Aim to work up to 12 Sun Salutes (six reps each side!). I love this workout as it energises and activates the body, especially the natural rhythms and peristalsis of the body. It helps to eliminate toxins. The body is bent forwards and backwards and this really benefits the spine, helping to bring a fresh supply of blood and oxygen to the whole body and internal organs. Wonderful!

Here is a brief introduction to the sequence for Sun Salutation. This is a basic sequence and there are many variations. Practice carefully remembering when to breathe in and when to breathe out; in time it will become second nature. (If you cannot manage to go into push up position as at position 6, just drop to knees as you are still exhaling, forehead to floor then push the upper body/torso through the hands. There are other alternatives to this for beginners so please ask your teacher for advice and demonstration). As you build up your arms you may then attempt to do the full position as in 6).

Remember start slowly; as you practice and become more familiar then the flexibility will follow.

ROUND 1—LEFT LEG

(The photos will assist you)

1. Begin with feet naturally apart, hands together, breathing naturally.

2. INHALE, stretching upward and backward, energising the body.

3. EXHALE, bending down, as you reach for the toes, touching if you can, bend knees if necessary, just hanging there allowing the back to stretch and open.

4. INHALE, **LEFT LEG** moves backward, right knee bent, as you are now lunging and looking forward, hands on floor, by knees supporting your weight, looking forward still, strong posture

5. EXHALE, right leg joins left leg, feet hip width apart, pressing heels into floor, you are now in an INVERTED V SHAPE, emphasis on pushing buttocks up to the ceiling, opening up, hands firm pressed into floor, arms straight, opening the shoulders wide, allow the head to relax, just hanging, no tension, allow the shoulders to open up, wide, not restricted, the heels do not need to be on floor, just stretch the hamstring, feel it opening. This is DOWNWARD DOG, as you continue with the exhalation try and press heels to floor but not necessary if only

beginner, flexibility will come with practice. (5 & 6 are fluid quick motions as are all the sun salute movements but again the fluidity will come in time).

6. Continue with EXALATION as you drop to knees, push torso through arms, dropping hips to floor, front of body stretched and open, shoulders dropped and passive, don't hunch, looking forward, neck soft, head lifted, this is COBRA, very energising for whole of spine! (Make the exhalation last for 4—6 counts).

   (The breath here is important, exhaling whilst you move into COBRA as you bring up the body into COBRA begin to INHALE).

7. INHALING now as you rest in COBRA, looking forward for count of 2.

8. EXHALING now as you return to DOWNWARD DOG, from COBRA, lift body back onto knees, sit back on heels then push up into DOWNWARD DOG, hold posture, still breathing out.

9. INHALE, bringing left leg under body, back into lunge as you look, forward, strong postures as in (4) above.

10. EXHALE, Right leg moves up to meet Left leg, return to touch toes (UTTANASANA) as in (3) above.

11. INHALING, Return to position 2 above.

12. Return to position (1)

REPEAT ABOVE PROCESS NOW BUT THIS TIME BRINGING THE RIGHT LEG FORWARD AS IN (4) ABOVE AND FINISHING AS IN (12) ABOVE. THIS COMPLETES ONE ROUND. YOU CAN WORK ON 3—4 ROUNDS AS LONG AS YOU USE BOTH LEFT AND RIGHT LEGS. THIS BALANCES OUT THE BODY. FINISH OFF IN CORPSE POSE, AND RELAX FOR 3—5 MINUTES, LISTENING TO THE BREATH, ALLOWING THE BODY, PULSE, HEART AND MIND TO ENJOY THIS EXPERIENCE.

The images show me taking the left leg back. As I come back to the final picture I will begin again, this time taking the right leg back. Always start at the top left corner of your Yoga mat. The final picture, with me in prayer position is shown slightly differently as I wanted to show you how to finish. You will finish top left of the mat as in the beginning image. Work with the breath, slowly and controlled. If you are bending over, exhale, if you are opening up inhale. This is very invigorating and a TOTAL BODY WORKOUT....enjoy!

SUN SALUTES ROUTINE:

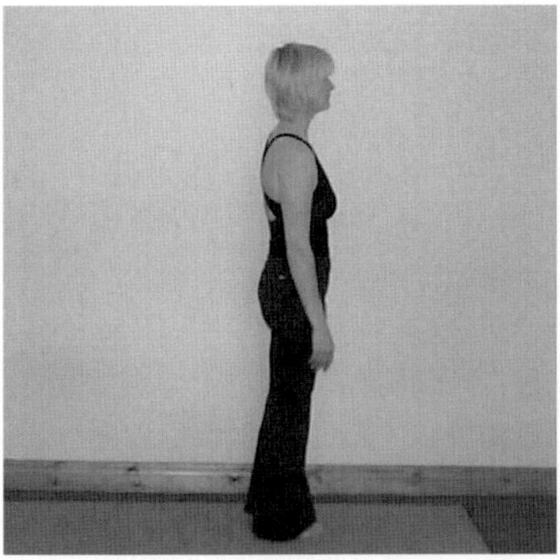

Pose 1

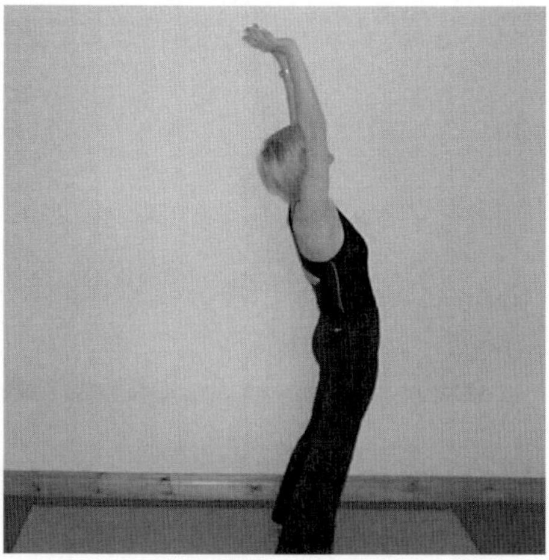

Pose 2

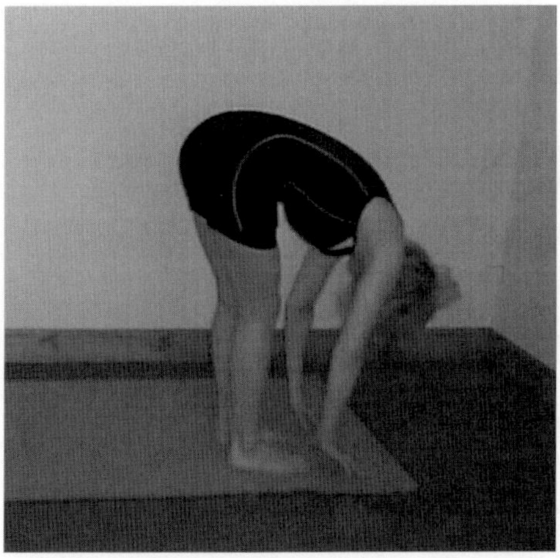

Pose 3

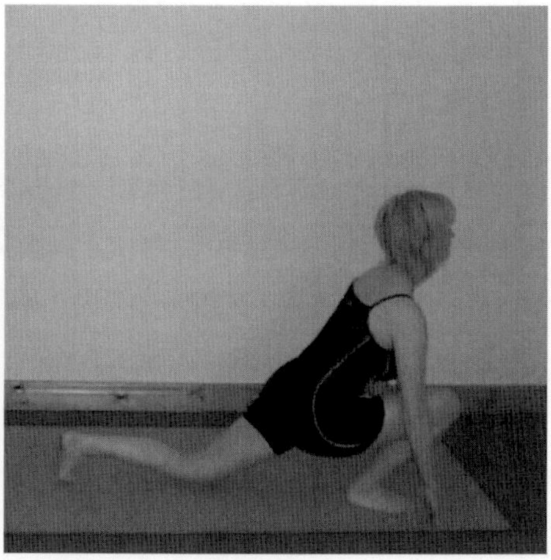

Pose 4

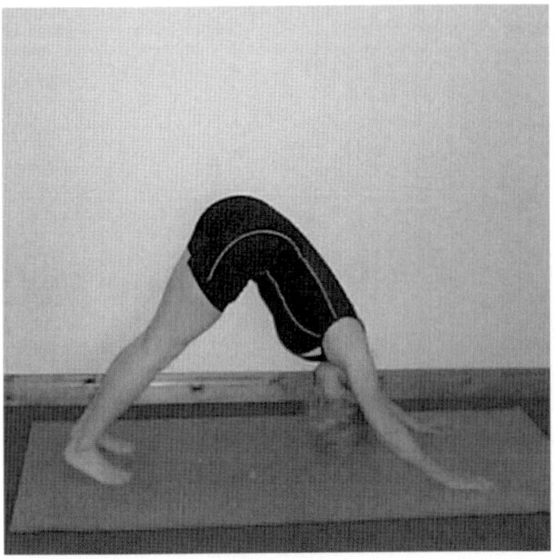

Pose 5

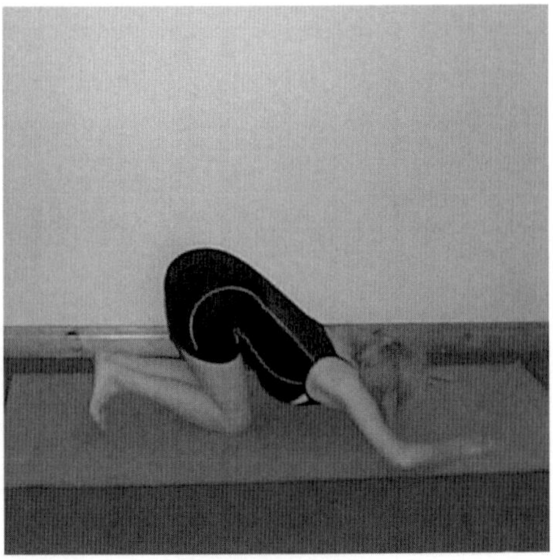

Pose 6

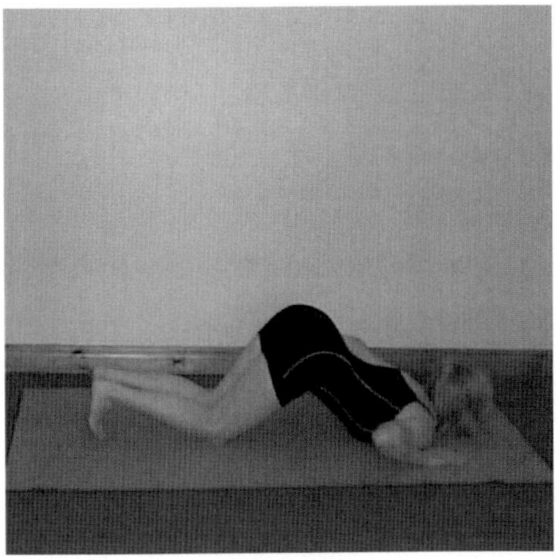

Pose 7

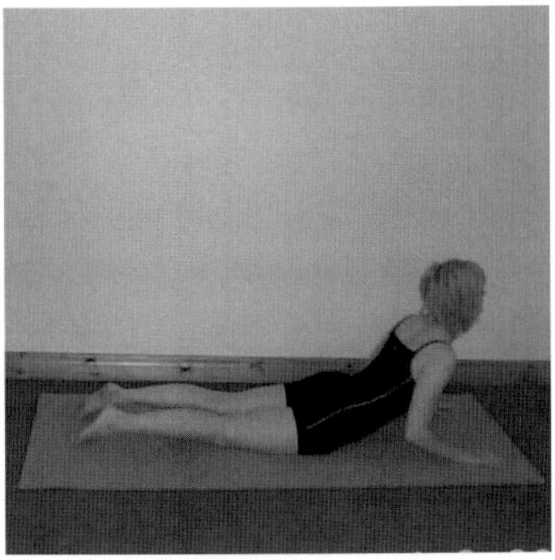

Pose 8

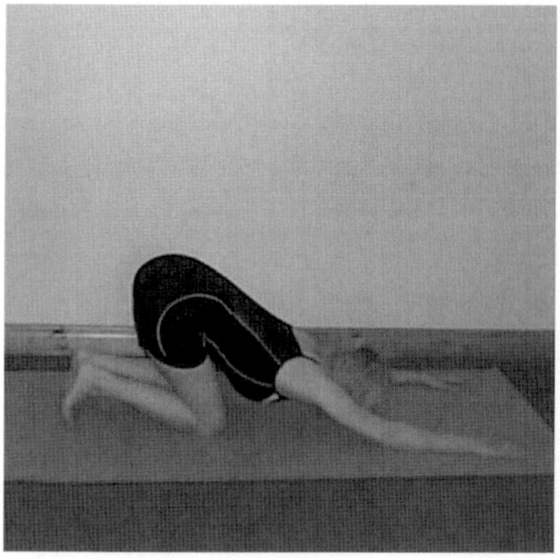

Pose 9

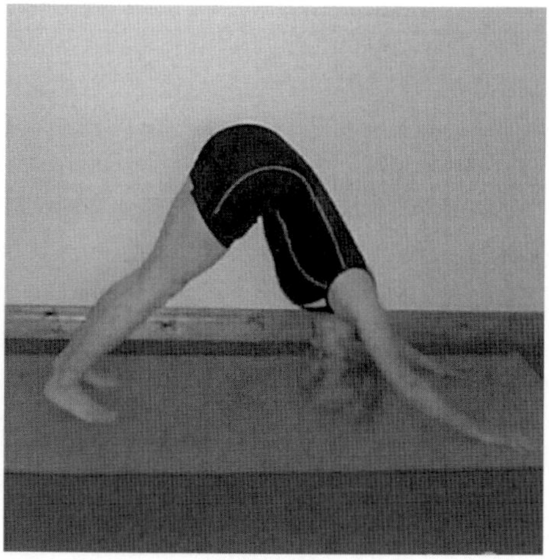

Pose 10

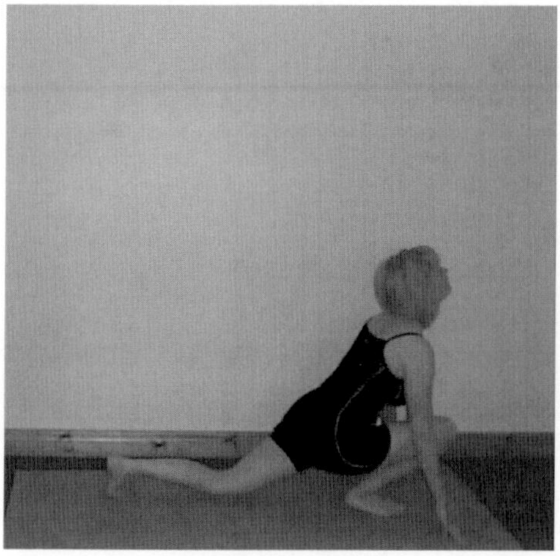

Pose 11

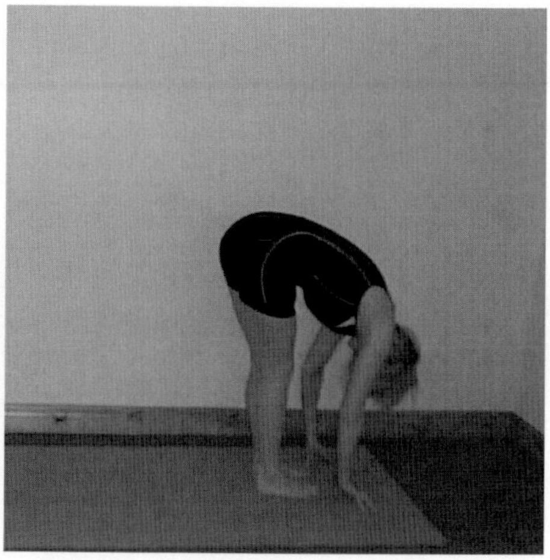

Pose 12

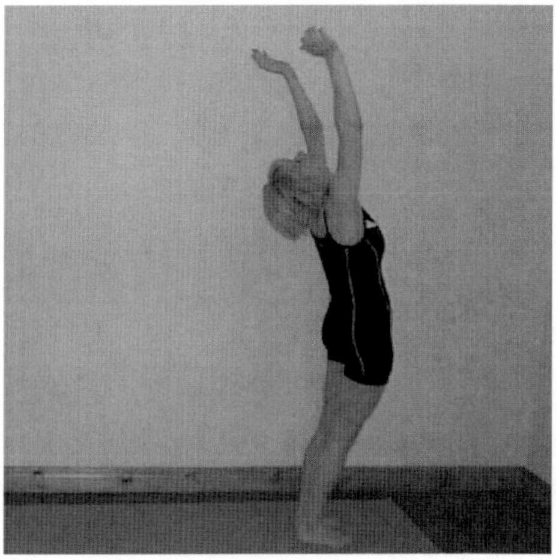

Pose 13

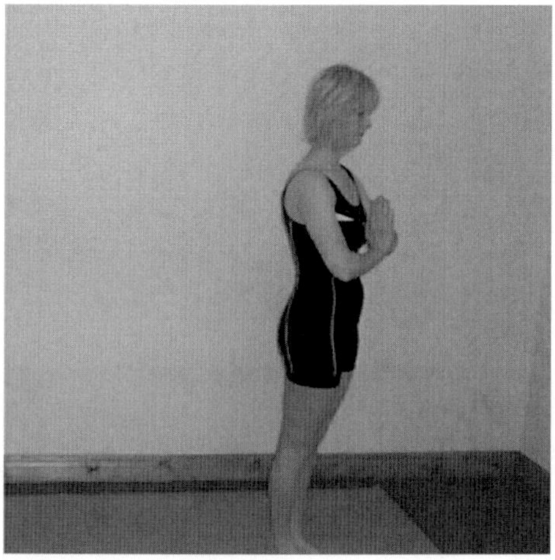

Pose 14

(Now repeat all images taking the right leg back)

SECTION 12
SELF-HEALING TECHNIQUES

We all have the amazing ability to heal ourselves. Over thousands of years this art of self-healing has been lost. I am going to attempt to invite you to bring this back into your life again. We actually see evidence of self-healing every day of our lives. When a child falls over what does the Mother do, she will place her hand on the child where he/she has fallen. If we bang our arm or our head or have a pain, we immediately take our hand to that area of the body. What do you do if you have a headache, you take your hands up there and hold your head, you hurt your knee, hand, elbow etc, the action is relatively the same, we reach for the spot with our hands. This is comforting but also is an instinctive action of healing.

One great technique to bring us back in touch with ourselves is to lie down and to place one hand on the heart centre and one on the solar plexus, lower abdomen. This firstly brings us in touch again with ourselves but also offers comfort by just the simple act of placing on of hands, our own hands. Holding the hands there you can say something like "I am now healed and comforted, I offer love to my heart and comfort to my soul" or words to that effect. Just spending this quiet time for 5—10 minutes with yourself can work wonders.

There is also the art of Reiki Healing. I am a Reiki Healer and have found this to be a remarkable tool in assisting with Endo pain management. It first of all calmed me down to the point where I felt more in control of my life and felt more balanced and complete. It is a simple and wonderful tool that you can use and if you so choose you can go on to use it to heal others.

There are two ways to receive Reiki. One way is to go and have the treatment as a client; the other is to become attuned to the Reiki energies. It is up to you and I am in no way urging everyone to go out and become a Reiki healer! It is your choice but I will say that this is one tool that I could not live without. Read books on it and familiarise with what it is all about. It is not everyone's cup of tea, as many don't understand how the energies work. Make your own decision. You can find out about local healers in your area from surfing the net or in your local telephone directory.

There are also different types of Reiki but they basically serve the same purpose, healing through universal energy. There are some very good books on the subject if you wish to read and familiarise yourself with this unique healing art before you consider trying it for yourself. You will love it, I'm sure of that. Visit your local bookstore and look in the Complementary/Alternative/Mind/Body/Spirit sections. They should stock a good variety of Reiki books as it is becoming very popular.

Your own Personal Inner Healer

As a spiritual healer I often use techniques that require me to go within myself and bring calm and tranquillity to my life, so important in this busy world today! For instance there is an unusual technique you can utilise which I again have personally found very beneficial. It involves lying down in a comfortable position and then taking a journey inside of your body. Here's how it's done and you can adapt this method to however you want to work.

Finding a comfortable lying down position (ideally Corpse pose as shown in the Yoga section).

Begin with relaxing the body; focusing on the breath as you inhale the stomach rises, as you exhale the stomach falls, focusing on this movement of the breath as you allow the body to relax further. I would like to add here that some of you might find this bizarre but give it a go, you might be pleasantly surprised. It is also very useful this practice as it gives us time to ourselves and to get in contact with ourselves as in this day and age we do lose contact with who we are and it is very important that we spend time nurturing and loving our inner self. This is when healing begins to take place on a subconscious level. When we are relaxed and in a state of meditation as you will be when doing practices such as this one, our body and mind rest and we switch off the outside world.

Lets begin:

When you are ready, eyes gently shut, imagine in your mind's eye that you have a little helper inside of you, this can be anyone you like person, animal. I use a little cartoon fellow with a white doctors jacket its really up to you so use your imagination and be sure to see it/him/her clearly. When you have this pictured in your mind's eye you then begin on your inner journey. Scanning your body for any areas of discomfort and you take your awareness to that area and use your little helper. For example:

If you suffer from Asthma, you can visualise this little helper inside the lungs, brushing them down and cleansing each lung. Imagine him bringing in fresh air, fresh energy and giving your lungs a spring clean! Your imagination is the key here and use whatever methods you like. With Endo I use the following techniques but again its entirely up to you but here is a little of what I use:

I imagine my helper inside my abdomen, close to my ovaries and other surrounding organs/tissues. I imagine him giving out bright golden light from his hands that surround my organs and cleanse and revitalise every membrane, every cell, and every part of me from the waist down. (It may help if you look at pictures of the body organs so you can picture clearer, but this is not really necessary).

I then imagine him with a hose and from that hose comes sparkling silver water of the purest kind and I allow that water to wash over me and cleanse every part of me. You can use this technique for any organ, any part of you where you feel discomfort. Each person will be different and you will know which areas of the body you choose to work with. Don't be afraid to experiment. It's really fun! For the heart centre, emotions and tightness in the chest I find that using pink, green and white colour/energies really help. You can also use affirmations such as "with this pink/green/white colour I now strengthen my heart and emotions and allow the negative energies to release as I exhale.

Experiment. There are no boundaries and this is your own personal physician! With severe pain you can imagine your little helper massaging the area/organ/tissue and releasing the pain, or imagine him with a golden torch that he shines on the pain and it disperses. It's all to do with imagination and how you want to work but I have personally found this very helpful. In times of great stress, again lying down relaxing, eyes gently shut, imagine the hands of angels at your shoulder, placing their hands on you and from their hands there is a glowing healing light, allow this light to wash over you and sigh out all the tension. It really is up to you how you want to work and our imagination and beliefs can be our greatest friend.

A COLD SHOWER

I was introduced to this technique about 18 months ago whilst receiving some Bowen Technique Therapy in North Yorkshire. The lady gave me a talk about the healing properties of water and especially that of a cold shower. Briefly, our bodies are made up of about 80% water (forgive me if not exactly spot on here!) but basically we are made up mainly of water, blood, and fluid. Our bodies hold onto emotions, feelings, both past and present and these can manifest into physical Illness and disharmony within our body. Our Aura also holds a great deal of negativity, old patterns etc, and a cold shower is an amazing tool as it works on the Aura and cleanses it.

Here's what to do:

Begin initially with the water at a temperature you would normally shower in. Then slowly begin to turn the water to cold. Standing under the cold water for 5—10 seconds initially. The shiver feeling and the 'shock' gasp etc, is actually your aura cleansing itself. Releasing the negative energies that your body has been holding onto through the aura. This negativity penetrating and entering the body as just that—negativity and often Illness. Start of with 5—10 seconds initially. Allow the water to go over the front of the body then the back, and the head. Not too long on the head area just a second or two. Finish with the water a little warmer so you warm up the body.

Notice how you feel after the 'shock'. I personally find it kind of makes me forget how I felt when I first got into the shower. It is excellent for clearing up a foggy head too! As you get used to the cold water, shock and shivers you will begin to enjoy this shower. The important thing to remember is that shiver you feel; it is doing you the world of good. Notice how you feel after 3 –4 goes. I am sure you will see and feel the benefits for yourself and your body will love it. You can do this morning or evening. You can do it first thing to start the day and last thing at night. Cleansing and revitalising in the morning, preparing for bed and washing away the day in the evening.

This water therapy can have an almost immediate cleansing affect. Try it over a period of 1 week and see how you feel. Again, you will need to learn to tune into yourself, remember that quiet time I mentioned. Taking time to '*notice*' will require you to calm down and relax and tune in to your body. This is very important.

SECTION 13
DIET & NUTRITION

I guess a lot of you are fed up with being told that "you should eat this" and "not eat that" and "too much of that will kill you". The truth is we can all eat what we want in moderation and the key is to try and eat a balanced and varied diet and include vitamins, minerals, proteins and amino acids as these are the building blocks to good health. Sometimes we eat things because we like the taste but our body can suffer afterwards. We need to begin to recognise what foods benefit us and what foods do not. Here I have outlined just a few tips that have helped me. It is not saying they will assist you but read on and see what you think. A lot of it is common sense but I do feel some people eat a lot of things that really don't help the body. The body works hard to digest certain foods, too many additives, junk food etc. When we have Endometriosis we have to be kind to our body and give it food and fuel that is easy to digest and uncomplicated. Keep it simple, fruit is a good friend, fresh food and plenty of water. If you want to be naughty and treat yourself do so but in moderation and try and balance the diet out so you eat a variety of foods.

For example I try to keep away from fizzy drinks because they are full of E numbers and other chemicals that can give me an instant headache. I have learned over the years through keeping a food diary and recognising how I feel after certain foods, what doesn't suit me. There is an easier way and that is to take a food allergy test but then you end up with a list eliminating things you do like! I have found it more beneficial to keep to a routine diet, that is foods that I can tolerate but at the same time enjoy eating.

We are what we eat and if we take a little time to see exactly what we are eating, maybe we can educate ourselves as to what our bodies do and don't like rather than what is good and what is not good for us. Here are a few tips on diet for Endo sufferers. This list will vary according to each individual but if you adhere to it you might find that your symptoms are lessened by not drinking too much coffee or switching to decaff etc. I often meet people whom I know have not been well. When you ask them how they are doing they are 'still the same'. The next question I ask is 'have you made any changes to your lifestyle, diet, exercise etc' the answer is more often than not 'No'! How can you possible change if you are not willing to initiate the process.

If you are not willing to make an effort and try new things then you may have to continue to experience the same old symptoms. Dare to be different and see how you feel. After all we are what we eat and if we fill our body with junk food and food lacking in energy then we cannot expect to function at our best. Here are a few items to consider:

- Avoid too many 'e' numbers in food. Endo tends to make us a little foggy headed and the 'E' numbers will just add to this foggy feeling and fill our body with substances that are often toxic and our body cannot digest/eliminate these easily.

- Look at the ingredients when you buy things. If you see too many numbers and long words on the back you can bet it is full of gunge that you don't really want to have in your body. KEEP IT SIMPLE, the fewer simpler ingredients that you can understand are going to be of benefit and not clog up your guts!

- Fizzy Drinks—ok in moderation but if a drink contains ingredients such as nutrasweet or Aspartame etc this converts to formaldehyde in the body (formaldehyde is what they use to preserve dead bodies with!) so say no more. Try and drink more natural fruit juices and read the label, the more natural the label the better the drink is for you. You are what you eat/drink.

- Apple Juice—Again use the more natural apple juices and not the 'concentrated' kind. Many supermarkets sell fruit juices and label them as 'natural and fresh' when they are actually concentrated. The more natural and 'live' juices will have a very short expiry date so opt for these. Concentrated Apple juice is also high in sugar content, which can feed bacteria and won't help those who suffer from Candida/Thrush, which are very common with Endometriosis. This type of sugar can also deplete adrenal levels so think of your body before you consume too many sugary drinks, and always opt for the freshly squeezed variety.

- Chocolate and sweets—many people crave sweet things. In moderation they are ok but they do contain sugar and the body works hard to break this down. Some of it is converted into energy but the more natural sugars such as those obtained from fruits are better for you and more easily digested. They don't add to your hips and thighs either!

- Eat lots of vegetables—try ones you haven't had before. Remember what you put in your body is going to help you. One of my favourites is Squash with a little sunflower oil/extra virgin olive oil. You might want to add some to your daily diet. The body loves the bright colours of the food. Its good to remember that whatever you put in your mouth has to be digested so try and eat simple foods and chew it well. If you eat toffees, mars bars etc your body has to digest this and it can use up a lot of energy so try and eat foods that are easy to digest.

- Dairy—limit your dairy intake. Too much of it is not good for you and I personally found that going to Goats milk instead of cow's really eased a lot of symptoms such as bloated stomach, gas, fuzzy head, sinus problems, groggy feeling. I also lost a little more weight not having cows milk so another added benefit. We don't actually need milk. As babies we need it but as adults it really does not benefit us. Yes you get calcium but you can also get calcium from cheese and vitamin/mineral supplements. There are lots of alternatives on the market today and many of the major supermarkets sell alternatives to dairy products. The taste may be unfamiliar to start with but you will soon get used to it. If you cannot give dairy up altogether try and alternate. Dairy products cause a great deal of allergies and people have found through eliminating dairy from diet many symptoms such as bloating, constipation, sinus congestion to name but a few clear up after a few weeks. Dairy products also contain calories so you may find you lose a little weight to boot!

- Cheese—cheese is ok. It gives us protein. Although I am not a cheese lover I try and have a few pieces each week for the calcium content.

- Organic—I must admit I do buy a lot of organic products and yes I do believe they work for me, but it is a personal choice. Organic stuff tends to have fewer chemicals.

- Prune Juice is excellent for the intestines and for our natural rhythm! A glass of prune juice is equal to one portion of fruit a day and keeps you regular.

- Bread—Bread contains Yeast, and if you have Endo you may also have Thrush and or Candida to which I will say leave bread well alone or use a more organic type, which you can buy. Many of us bloat after eating bread and this is the gas being produced and the body trying to digest it. Ryvita are a safe alternative or more natural breads with less yeast. I have known people lose a lot of weight through eliminating bread from their diet and they don't really miss it. If you have to eat bread try the more natural breads, the wholemeal, seeded loaf. Wholemeal is better for you because of the fibre content and you can buy some breads that have sunflowers etc in them. These are really good for you. Remember I am not a Dietician or a Nutritionalist, I just learned from adapting my diet to how my body feels.

- Salad—you can never eat too much salad. Again it is the colours and the freshness that is the key here. Red onions in abundance as these are good for the heart and blood. Might want to carry a pack of mints round with you after though!

- Chicken—love chicken and I tend to steam it rather than fry it or put it in oven. Steaming food keeps it in a more natural state and I personally feel it tastes better. You don't get too much of the fat either. Chicken is however, pumped with additives and hormones and these do not help Endo sufferers or anyone come to think of it. So again, limit your intake, you don't have to stop altogether or turn veggie! But just limit what you eat and vary it. Buy organic if you can. The Chinese actually cook their chicken in boiling water, flash boil, it tastes divine. Again each to their own but don't be afraid to experiment with cooking. The less time it takes to prepare the better it is going to be for you. No messing around, simple food. Not too many additives etc. Since writing this I have learned from my Naturopath that Chicken can contain a lot of virus. I have since opted to limit my intake. These virus can cause colds, flu symptoms and make us feel lowsy, and eating such foods as chicken, veal, pork, bacon etc can, over a long period of time cause us many problems. This includes organic meats. I am really cutting down and I advise you try Tofu as a substitute a few times a week. Of course, it's up to you, each to their own!

- Junk food—in moderation. We don't want to be too healthy! but at the same time limit your intake. A little of what you fancy does you good but I don't think any junk food really benefits us. It's very fattening to. Remember that the more complicated our food, i.e. the more ingredients that are in it the harder our system has to work to digest it. Take it easy and be kind to yourself. Junk food has lots of additives and E numbers that our body finds hard to digest sometimes so take things easy.

- Fruit—melons, apples, oranges, grapefruit, grapes, etc very good for you but fruit diets are really bad for you. They stir up toxins in the blood stream, which can make you have headaches, joint ache, upset tummy etc. Fruit should be eaten alone away from meals so snack on them in between main meals/30 minutes before and 3 hours after a meal. This will give the body time to digest the main foods otherwise the fruit begins to ferment in the stomach and causes gas and bloating.

- Water—very good for you. The body is made up of 80% water and through exercise, stress, working etc we use up a great deal and often suffer from dehydration. Drinking a couple of glasses of water throughout the day helps to stop this dehydration and also aid digestion and stop constipation. Try this in the morning: organic lemon cut up and added to a cup of hot water, it's a great start to the day and it converts to alkaline in the body which heals and soothes our internal organs.

- Smoothies—I love smoothies and juicing. You can put anything you like in them. A favourite of mine is: strawberries, banana, raspberries and apple juice. Juice it and drink it, lovely and a quick vitamin fix. If you are one of these people who can't stomach anything in the morning try a smoothie or juice some fruit. Our bodies need something in the morning and this is light and gives us lots of energy.

- Sugars—refined sugars such as those we use daily for baking, tea and coffee cause fluctuations in our blood sugars. The body goes on a high when it has sugar and then hits a low craving more buzz from the sugars. There are four supplements that you can take to help balance out sugar metabolism if you are worried that you may be taking too much sugar.

L-glutamine—an amino acid shown to prevent the development of glucose regulating problems. A rat study examining the effects of L-glutamine on blood glucose regulation found the addition of a 2% L-glutamine infusion to rats' diets prevented any change in the rats plasma glucose and insulin levels.

Chromium Picolinate is a mineral that helps regulate blood sugar levels. In a recent study 180 men and women with Type II Diabetes were divided into three groups each supplemented twice daily with either 100-mcg-chromium piconliate, 500-mcg-chromium picolinate place or a placebo. They maintained their existing diets and lifestyles. After four months, glucose levels were significantly reduced in the 500-mcg group, while insulin values ere significantly reduced in both chromium groups.

Gymnema Sylvestrea is an Indian Ayurvedic herb commonly used by Diabetics. Animal tests and test tube studies suggest that Gymnema extracts suppress intestinal absorption of saccharides, which prevents blood sugar elevations. A 1997 Japanese animal study of Gymnemic acids from GF. Sylvestre leaves looked at the effects of the acids on blood glucose in guinea pigs and rats. The acids suppressed the elevation of blood glucose by inhibiting glucose uptake in the intestine (*extract taken from Journal of Veterinary Medical Science, 1997, vol 59*).

Alpha Lipoic acid—one of the most potent antioxidants to date, has been the subject of studies investigation its ability to improve glucose utilisation and improve nerve Illness caused by diabetes. In patients with Type II Diabetes, alpha-lipoic acid increased muscle cell glucose uptake and increased insulin sensitivity (*extract taken from Diabetes 1999, vol 48*).

Making better food choices can solve most blood sugar problems. For example complex carbohydrates—such as those found in beans, fruits and vegetables—are digested more slowly, thus providing a more sustained sugar supply. When you have a meal try and let the body digest it. We all too often eat, get up and get on with something else, this disturbs the body's digestive process and we often end up with indigestion. Sit for 30 minutes after a meal or take things easy thus allowing your body to do its natural functions in peace.

Your body can only run on what you have put into it. If you balance your diet and eat quite healthily then you can't go far wrong. One thing I do that does help me is that one day a week, say Saturday I will have a juice in the morning then nothing till the evening. Giving myself a 6—7 hour break from eating. Not to lose weight, although it does help! But to give my system a rest. You may experience a slight headache and a little nausea this is usually the time to have something to eat. Avoid too much salt and too much sweet stuff. If you want sweet go for the more natural alternatives such as fruit bars or just plain old fruit. The more natural the better for you. Try and incorporate into your diet fibre, organic short grain brown rice and Physillium husks. Not all three! But introducing these to your diet will help the elimination process and this stops toxins and waste building up in the colon which can make us feel ill, sluggish and bloated.

I do find with Endo that I can't leave it too long between meals. If you find yourself getting dizzy because you haven't eaten then try and carry a snack such as an apple, orange or organic rice cakes to nibble on or when you feel your body needs it. If you eat three balanced meals a day you may not need to snack.

Indigestion

Many Endo sufferers complain of Indigestion. We don't all have it but at least you can rest assured that you are not alone with this and there are probably 100s of women out there who suffer from the same feeling after a meal. Ginger helps a great deal. Try and include some in your diet, or just as a hot drink, cut up and bash a little ginger (it is in the bashing that the juices are released and you get the best benefit!). Pop a little in a cup and pour on boiling water. It really is a wonderful tonic. Use it in stir-fries and curries and pep up a salad with a few pieces of bashed ginger. Great for sore throats and when you feel a little run down. Magnesium is also beneficial. If you don't like to take this orally in tablet form, try adding some Epsom salts to your bath. Charcoal tablets are a must for Indigestion. I have been taking them for the past 12 months on the onset of indigestion and the charcoal has a very calming affect on the abdomen. Indigestion symptoms are gone within about 10 minutes of taking the tablets. The Charcoal soaks up the air bubbles that cause the indigestion and they are very natural. You can buy these from most High Street Health Stores. Charcoal really does help for menstrual pain also as a lot of this is down to too much gas!

Tea/Coffee/ Herbal teas

I drink coffee both caff and decaff. What I will say is that caffeine will add to the mind chatter and buzzy/fuzzy head thing we often get with Endo. Try and substitute caffeine for Decaff but remember you can get withdrawal symptoms from reducing your caffeine intake. Do it in moderation then it won't be too much of a shock to the system. Herbal teas help. With the indigestion try peppermint tea. It calms the digestive tract and helps the stomach. Herbal teas are great for bedtime. Chamomile, Valerian or Lime flower teas help us to relax and aid a restful nights sleep.

Cranberry Juice:

Take note of this one. If you don't include it in your diet then do! It is fantastic for Urinary Tract Infections such as Cystitis and Thrush. I drink gallons of it and can say hand on heart that I don't get either of these symptoms anymore. Try it hot before bed, lovely! You can also buy Cranberry supplements. These work to and are very gentle with no side effects.

Amino Acids

Amino Acids are basically the building blocks of the body. Besides building cells and repairing tissue, they form antibodies to combat invading bacteria & viruses; they are part of the enzyme & hormonal system; they build nucleoproteins (RNA & DNA); they carry oxygen throughout the body and participate in muscle activity. When protein is broken down by digestion the result is 22 known amino acids. Eight are essential (cannot be manufactured by the body) the rest are non-essential (can be manufactured by the body with proper nutrition). So you can see from this brief overview just how important a role these little fellows play in our health.

I wanted to include a little bit about these and their importance as I have been taking a naturopathy programme for the past 14 months, which involves a drink that contains various Amino Acids. The results have been remarkable and this has highlighted to me what an important role these Amino Acids play in our overall health and well-being. Some amino acids can be obtained from the food we eat but not all. It is therefore necessary to take them from another source, usually in a powdered form. A website that gives more information regarding a Naturopathy Programme that included Amino Acids is **www.onlinenaturopath.net**. These people are pioneers in what they are doing and anyone interested in taking the programme should contact them direct using the website.

If changing your diet and introducing new items you may want to keep a Food Diary. This is helpful if you are experiencing any dramatic symptoms. Maybe they occur after eating something. Jot down what you eat and how you feel immediately after, 2 hours after, 3 hours, etc.

I have included a table for you to use should you wish to do this. It may help you to eliminate things from your diet that your body does not like. I could talk forever about food, what to eat, what not to eat but this would be mostly what I have found works for me. The basic principals of eating are what you need to stick to. Keep it fresh, colourful, balanced and tasty. Introduce new ingredients and experiment. The fresher you eat the healthier you will be. I have attached a sample Food Diary Monitor Sheet towards the end of the book for you to use if you wish.

SECTION 14
MONITORING YOUR PROGESS & KEEPING A DIARY:

Beginning the healing process may be a long haul. Start by tuning into your body, noticing, feeling, listening to how you feel, what symptoms you have, write them down if you wish. I am a firm believer of connecting with our own bodies and feeling grounded helps us to stay in control of our bodies. Sometimes this illness can be very complicated with many different symptoms. Try to tune in to them one by one; for example:

- Stomach cramps
- Hot sweats
- Backache
- Headache
- Cramps
- Bloated
- Overactive mind
- Depression
- Hot
- Cold
- Sweaty
- Pain

Open up a diary of how to deal with the pain. As you practice Yoga, self-healing, new diet, elimination of certain foods etc, write down and monitor how you feel.

Use the following table to keep a record of how you feel. You don't have to do it religiously everyday but initially use it and see how you go. If you find something is particularly helping you then keep it up and pass it on to your friends.

SYMPTOMS MONITORING SHEET

Date	Symptoms before activity	Activity	Symptoms post activity
01/01/03	Sore stomach, leg cramps, bloated	Fruit diet, plenty of water, went for walk round block	Felt better after walk, don't feel all bloated as have given stomach a rest. Feel more energy after going walking
03/01/03 06/01/03	Headache, heaviness in stomach, feel bit depressed Depressed, tension in shoulders, cracking headache, No Aspro!	Did 20 minutes of Yoga, energising routine* followed by relaxation and breathing for 10 minutes. Had hot bath, tuned into my body and began relaxing in the bath, breathing routine, neck rolls and 10 minutes yoga.	Feel much better, headache gone, feel as if mood has lifted slightly. Must remember those postures! The breathing helped loads! I could feel my muscles relaxing from the hot bath, and the breathing helped to unwind me. Headache easing off a bit especially after neck rolls, could feel energy block lifting as I released my neck muscles and released the tension. Will do that again!
8 Jan 2003	Stomach Cramps and bloated again	Cut down on my coffee/tea substituted for decaff and had a couple of herbal teas. Drank a few glasses of cranberry juice. Went for a swim.	Swimming helped a lot. It got me out the house for a bit and was quite energising! Not much of a swimmer but I think it gave me that little boost I needed, plus have done some exercise which helps. The cranberry juice seems to have helped a little with the stomach cramps. Have had a bit of a headache with the decaff but will persevere.
12/01/03	Slight headache but not as bad as before. Legs ache after swimming	Still taking cranberry juice, had a walk in the park and came back, hot shower and did some visualisation/meditation for 10 minutes.	3 days without coffee, feeling a little less highly strung! Stomach much better and the fruit has helped. Also taking the water has stopped a few of the niggly headaches I have been getting. Don't feel too bad today at all. Starting to be more positive. The visualisation seems easier as not having so much coffee. Seems to be easier to relax more.

These are a few examples of what you might want to put. Use anything you like. Remember the 'tuning in' learn to 'know' how you feel. The noticing of the subtle differences that can occur. Do yourself a favour and give yourself the valued time out it needs if it is only 15—20 minutes, twice a week meditation or using yoga or the visualisation techniques.

You will be amazed how just getting to know you from the inside out will create major changes for you in mind body and spirit. I am not a doctor but someone who took a stand to take an interest in her own health. To educate myself with Western and Eastern Therapies and with ways that can enhance our health, mind, body and spirit through the use of postures and other simple techniques that don't cost the earth. Relaxing the body and taking time for yourself is a great healing tool in itself and it's free. Yoga is a therapy that is tried and tested and has proven very beneficial over the years to help many people from all walks of life, all shapes, ages and sizes.

SECTION 15
ALTERNATIVE PRODUCTS

The products mentioned here are not offered as a cure for Endometriosis but are listed to assist you. With so many products on the market today we often don't know what is good and what is not, what works and what doesn't so I have listed a few here. If trying anything new please consult your GP. It is all about finding a balance and each and everyone of us are unique and this is important to remember. There are so many of us with drastically different symptoms to numerous to mention here but the point I am making is that it is your personal journey, to find out what helps you with your specific symptoms.

Maximol Solution

(Neways International) A mineral supplement full of trace minerals that our body needs.

I have used this for 4 years now and have felt many benefits. It has particularly helped me with weight management, energy, fatigue, period pains, and headaches and seems to support the body in many ways. Those people that I know who have used this rate this product very highly. You can order this from Neways website and can call Neways to find out about distributors in your area.

Mercy Oil

(www.mercyoilproducts.com)—A natural oil that is made from black cumin seeds and other ingredients. It can be purchased as a muscle rub, capsule form, drinking form and inhalant. It cleanses from the inside out so good for parasites in the digestive tract and bowel, and it can assist with Candida and Thrush, which often accompany Endo.

Omega 3 & Other Oils

Evening Primrose Oil*

Pumpkin Seed Oil*

Extra virgin olive oil (for cooking and as a dressing for salads/pasta. The Cold Pressed variety are the better ones to use. Try taking a teaspoon of this each morning.)

These oils really help to support the body. They are especially beneficial for nervous system, Eyes, skin, nails and hair and also benefit many internal organs. Omega 3 is good for the heart and lungs and the evening primrose is used by many women to support PMS and hormone function.

Cranberry (Juice or Capsules)

Taken each day are very beneficial for the Urinary tract. Cleansing and purifying the bladder, kidneys and ease symptoms associated with Cystitis. There are also products you can buy to support the reproductive system and bladder.

Epsom Salts—(Very valuable to know!)

Now here's a little gem. Try a tablespoon in your bath 4 days before the onset of the menses (your period!). It helps elimination of toxins, calms the heat in the body and stops headaches. Its something to do with the Magnesium and it's cooling effect. I also bath in this twice a week. I cannot remember the last time I had a headache. Headaches are often due to the body burning and friction and many of us suffer from headaches/heat when we are due our monthly bleed. Try it for a few weeks and see how it feels. I don't bathe without this now.

Walnuts

Try eating 6 walnuts a day. Walnuts are very beneficial. Walnuts can permeate almost anything and so when we digest them they cling on to toxins within the body and bring it out with them. They really help to regulate the bowels to!

Natural Progesterone Creams

Symptoms of PMS that respond to Natural Progesterone

Headache
Motor coordination
Migraines
Excess use of Alcohol
Epilepsy
Fainting spells
Lethargy
Leg and other muscle cramps
Eye irritation
Feeling of being crazy
Breast engorgement
Asthma
Backache
Cold extremities
Infertility
Fibrosis
White spots in fingernails
Capillary fragility
Toxaemia of pregnancy
Gall bladder symptoms
Frequent urination
Accident proneness
Falling hair
Lowered libido
Irritability
Depression
Mood swings
Other drug excess
Crying and weeping
Feeling of panic
Frustration
Blurred vision
Hot flashes
Night sweats
Memory difficulties
High stress
Weight gain
Sore throat
Runny nose
Stiffness

Hypoglycaemic reactions
Spontaneous abortion
Constipation, gas
Inflammatory diseases
Poor dream recall
Dry skin
Water retention
Hoarseness
Sinusitis
Upper respiratory complaints
Infections
Dry hair
Exhaustion - mental and physical
Attempted suicide
Aggression and violence
Self-inflicted injuries
Child abuse - verbal and physical
Sudden anger
Joint and muscle pain
Runny eyes
Fly and colds
Breast tenderness
Bruise easily
Herpes simplex
Joint swelling
Lack of appetite
Hysteria
Slow digestion
Insomnia
Inability to concentrate
Eye puffiness
Arthritis flare
Dark circles under eyes
Facial pallor
Greasy hair
Painful menses
Bloating
Boils

Although many ladies who have tried Natural Progesterone creams have found many benefits—if you are considering taking them for any of the above symptoms please consult your doctor first. It is advisable to have a hormonal blood test to assess the level of Oestrogen, adrenaline and Progesterone already present in the body. There are Natural creams containing Wild Yam, which, can help to alleviate some PMS/menopausal symptoms but again always consult your GP. Some of these symptoms won't just be down to PMS or Endometriosis and may be due to some other underlying cause so again see your GP and discuss with him/her how you feel. The advertisements on websites promoting these creams are all well and good but what works for one will not necessarily work for another. It is finding that all-important balance. If you overload on Progesterone for example you can do yourself a great deal of damage. These products are outlined as an alternative but you should always consult your GP before trying.

Phiten (Titanium) Cream

After recently taking up Wing Chun (Martial Arts) I went to an Exhibition at the NEC where I purchased some Phiten Water Cream. The cream was designed with athletes in mind and those who suffer from Arthritis and reoccurring pain in parts of the body. I had suffered from neck pains for many years. A great deal of tension is located in the neck area from poor posture, working at a computer all day, poor sleeping position etc. But a lot of pain in the neck area is linked to hormones and menstrual cycle. I am not an expert but from what I can understand from information received from a Naturopath is that the pain in the neck is due to activity that goes on in the brain, the Hypothalamus, when the body is preparing for menstruation. I never would have looked at the body in this way but it all works in unison and if something is not quite right then the body will show us pain.

The Phiten cream contains Titanium in a very natural form and I must say I used to have to sit with a hot water bottle and take 2 pain killers every 2—3 weeks but I don't get that pain any more. It seems to be the Titanium in the cream and it has a very relaxing affect. You can visit the site to read up about this product. I have highlighted the website at the end of the book.

NATUROPATHY—NATURE CURE CLINIC (AUSTRALIA)

I briefly mentioned earlier that I have recently started on a naturopathy programme, which involves taking 3 drinks each day made up from a number of bottles of ingredients, which contain a combination of amino acids, herbs, minerals and vitamins. This programme has been made up for my own individual requirements. The naturopath is Australian and you can find more about him and his unique programme by visiting www.onlinenaturopath.net. The programme is expensive but after being on it for 9 months I can honestly say that it is remarkable and my Endo symptoms have vanished. The programme works on rebuilding from within, our very core, the bone marrow, cells, muscles etc. I don't want to go into too much detail here as I believe that everyone should find out for themselves. What I will proudly say is that I have never felt so good, so balanced!

I have found improvement in many areas and can now report that I do not have any of the Endometriosis symptoms that I used to have. This programme teaches you about how we are at one with Nature. As I learn from Jeff Campbell in our monthly sessions how nature can provide us with a cure for many Illness. As with the brief explanation about my neck pain that I have given, I have learned how the body works, why pain occurs, what the reasons are behind the pain and it is very interesting. You learn to treat the 'cause' of the pain not just the 'symptoms'. I use castor oil packs and these are extremely beneficial.

Chemicals and toxins are around us day in day out. Our body absorbs a great deal of these toxins and chemicals and so it is no wonder we end up with Illness. The programme works to balance from the bone marrow, our very core, to our skin, hair, nails, organs, muscle tissue, every part of our very being is re-hydrated, rejuvenated—it is truly amazing (a word I don't use lightly but to be honest, it is the only word I can use to describe how I feel). My husband asked me the other day "how do you know you have cured your Endo!" my answer was simple "darling", I said "how do I know, I don't, all I do know is that I no longer have the symptoms". Simple enough answer, and very true.

As we are all unique individuals how therefore can we be given the same medication for the same Illness? This is something I could never understand and this is why I chose to go to the alternatives rather than conventional medicine. The programme works using nature to balance us from within. Treating the whole body, balancing and rejuvenating, releasing toxins that have been stored in the body for many years.

There is a form that you can fill out online whilst visiting the site and the Naturopath will contact you for a free consultation. The Naturopath, Jeff Campbell and his wife have worked for many years with Qualified Practitioners from all areas of medicine both conventional and alternative.

Our Monthly Cycle

Our monthly cycle is necessary for out body to release toxins and build up within our system. It is a natural occurrence and we should not interfere with this. (This is my own personal opinion). Many doctors and physicians, those who believe in the natural approach will agree with me here. Over the years we, as females, have learned to live with contraceptives in whatever form as a way of coping. It is not the answer. Masking the pain of Endometriosis and painful PMS is not the way forward. We may stop the pain, but what else is happening within our bodies? After being on this programme my system is free from any form of contraceptive.

I now feel completely natural and with my body rejuvenating thanks to the ingredients contained in the programme I feel a more natural woman and my periods are what I would class as normal, a natural occurring bodily function that doesn't hinder me like it used to. I am no longer sat on the loo for hours in agony. I no longer carry around the endless supply of tampons, sanitary towels and my handbag no longer resembles a pharmacy! What used to be a chore each month, facing my periods, dreading the week of pain and disruption, is now a breeze! I remember what my periods used to be like back in 1986 and realise that for years my body was working so hard to perform a natural function. I then interrupted this function with contraceptives, medication etc. No wonder I was having so many problems. The programme has given me a break. It has helped my body to perform this natural cycle once again with ease; naturally as it should be and the most wonderful feeling of all is that my system is toxin free. There are no words really to describe this feeling other than I feel all woman again.

This programme involves monitoring your health and symptoms from the first day you start the programme. It is very carefully designed for your own specific needs. I have found a great deal of benefits from being on this programme but again what suits one will not necessarily suit another. It is my wish that from reading the information contained in this book that you will see a different way of looking at your health. Whether you suffer from Endometriosis or just general discomfort during your menses, there are so many ways that you can help yourself. For me this programme has been the answer I was looking for.

I now have a regular as clockwork 4-day monthly bleed, no headaches and periods are bliss! I now look forward to actually having them, realising now that it is my body's way of releasing toxins, build up etc. We are at one with nature, our body is so closely linked with it but over the years we have lost this knowledge. If we begin to link ourselves in with the natural cycles this itself will hold many benefits. "No less than the trees and the stars you have a right to be here......"

SECTION 16
USEFUL WEBSITES

www.onlinenaturopath.net
www.helica.co.uk
www.shetrust.org.uk
www.mercyoilproducts.com
www.endouk.co.uk
www.healthypages.co.uk
www.simlynatural.org
www.worldofalternatives.com
www.soulworkers.co.uk
www.phiten.co.uk

SECTION 17

MY ENDO DIARY

Date	Activity	Symptoms before Activity	Symptoms post activity

<u>MY FOOD DIARY</u>

Date	What I ate Today	How I feel

SECTION 18
At One with Nature

I wanted to leave this to the very end. It is a very interesting fact and one that as time has gone by we have forgotten how very close to nature we really are. We are not just human beings existing but we are human beings existing on a planet and we belong to that planet. Our body is not just a body but part of the whole universe. Think of the sea, the waves how they time their rhythmic movements to the clouds, sun and moon. The shape of the earth, it is all interlinked and we are part of this great puzzle called life. As the leaves change in the autumn time, as the months bring with them different seasons, our body goes through a similar cycle, the cycle of life.

When you think of your monthly cycle don't think of it as a pain, as a hindrance, think of it as your 'nature cycle'. As the seasons change and move so does our body and as females our monthly cycle is part of this natural process. Each month our body goes through this cycle of cleansing, removal of toxins, preparing to conceive if we so wish. It is something that happens beyond our control and shows us how close to nature we are. Our monthly cycle is very closely linked to the cycle of the Moon. Our body works in harmony with Mother Nature.

I believe that illness occurs due to our body being out of sync with nature. Using medication can disturb our natural cycle; our body clock can become disturbed. Bringing back this natural balance through cleansing and rejuvenation in my opinion can help us to reclaim our health and bring balance to our mind, body and spirit.

Our monthly cycle starts off in the Pineal gland, which is situated inside our head, in the brain, behind the eyes. This tiny gland plays an important role in our monthly cycle and other body functions. It responds to light and darkness. For example how do you feel when you sit in the sun and your body quenches on the golden rays of the sun? you will love it, your body loves it, your mood lifts. Why do we all rush to go on holiday somewhere sunny? It is because we need and love the sun, not only to relax but our body needs the sun's energy. Sun beds are not the answer. I am talking of the natural rays from the sun. Looking towards the sun between the hours of 8am and 1pm in the afternoon with eyes closed will benefit you. The suns energies reach the pineal gland and we become energised. Think of a plant without the sun! it will wither and die. This is the same for us, not so severe I might add but it points out the importance of the Sun and how our bodies work with nature.

The Pineal Gland produces Melotonin which helps us to sleep at night. This little gland does not only register the amount of natural and artificial light we are exposed to daily but also alerts us with the changes in seasons throughout the year. We are so at one with nature and many of us don't realise. The Pineal Gland's main function is to alert the hypothalamus to begin the menstrual cycle. The hypothalamus itself is a very sensitive part of the endocrine system. This "blobby cluster" sits close to our emotional centre within the brain and can react adversely to emotional upheaval. When the hypothalamus is healthy it performs its duties quite well. When the hypothalamus is unbalanced and not performing properly it may give out incorrect signals to the Pituitary gland, causing this tiny gland to manufacture either too much or not enough hormones. This throws the body off balance.

One thing that can benefit you is to try the exercise given above. Looking towards the sun, eyes gently closed between 8am and 1pm (for about 5—10 minutes per day) will help your body to regain balance. If you can't see the sun or it is cloudy, look towards where the sun is hiding. This little trick is amazing, truly it is. Try it, it really boosts you and I find it helps to lift your mood.

Yoga is another way that we can jump start our natural cycle and bring back the natural rhythm as the postures work on the Endocrine system and many other systems within the body. There are many things you can do to help your body regain the balance it needs to perform the natural cycle with ease. It doesn't have to be complicated.

I have taken some information from a wonderful paper written by ***Linda Sparrowe.*** The Paper is called ***Menstrual Essentials*** and is an 8-page document outlining the Natural Cycle and how it works. I urge you to read this. It can be found at: www.thinkholistic.com/newspub/story.cfm?ID=44 visit the site and have a read. You will be enlightened I assure you.

I have crammed a lot into this little book. Don't feel that you have to go out and buy everything and try everything that is not what this book is for. It is hoped that you will take a little of what is shown here and try it. I have only shown what has worked for me and that I know has worked for others. There are a lot of old health secrets shown that have been lost over the years. Bring it back, educate yourself and learn. Keep it as simple and as natural as you can.

I do hope that you can learn to look at your health in a more natural way. If we give our body the right tools it will begin the natural healing process. Finding that all important inner harmony and balance is not so hard to attain.

With love and light

Tammy Lorraine Majchrzak